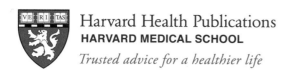

Dear Reader,

Most people take bladder and bowel control for granted—until something goes wrong. Then, unexpectedly, they find themselves hurrying to get to a bathroom on time, avoiding certain situations for fear of being embarrassed by bladder or bowel accidents, or relying on absorbent pads for protection. If you have had any of these experiences, you are not alone.

An estimated 20 million adults have urinary incontinence, and 19 million have fecal incontinence, with some experiencing both conditions. This unintended loss of urine or feces is significant enough to make it difficult for people to maintain good hygiene and carry on ordinary social and work lives. What's the cause? For women, it's typically a rarely discussed but common result of childbirth and aging. For men, it is often a prostate problem or a side effect of treatment for prostate problems.

Besides disrupting daily activities and nighttime sleep, incontinence can also chip away at your health. If you have stopped exercising for fear of leakage, for example, you are giving up one of the most effective strategies for maintaining health. In addition, getting up several times a night can lead to sleep deprivation. And incontinence that causes withdrawal from social interactions can contribute to depression.

Even more alarming, older people who frequently must rush to the bathroom are 45% more likely to fall, risking a fracture. Incontinence is also a leading cause of nursing home placement, and that prospect drives some people to try to hide their condition rather than seek help.

The good news is that treatments are becoming more effective and less invasive. For example, today's medications for urinary incontinence have fewer side effects than earlier ones. Exercises can help strengthen the muscles of the pelvic floor, shoring up those that control both bladder and bowel. Surgical options include less invasive outpatient procedures that can work as well as older, open surgical procedures.

Although incontinence can engender fear and embarrassment, rest assured that it is not a psychological problem or a personal failure. Incontinence is a medical symptom, and it deserves the same attention you would give to any other medical problem. This report describes the common causes of urinary and fecal incontinence for men and women and the treatments for these conditions.

Sincerely,

May M. Wakamatsu, M.D.
Medical Editor

Joseph A. Grocela, M.D.
Medical Editor

Liliana Bordeianou, M.D.
Medical Editor

Urinary incontinence

In the United States, an estimated four million men and 16 million women have moderate or severe urinary incontinence—the loss of reliable bladder control—and another 34 million feel the need to urinate with increasing urgency and frequency but manage to avoid accidents. Because damage sustained during vaginal childbirth is a major cause of incontinence, the problem is much more common in women, affecting more than 30% of those ages 70 and older (see Figure 1, below right). Men are less commonly affected—15% or more of those 70 and older, according to government estimates—but the rates are increasing as more men undergo surgery or other treatments of the prostate gland. More than half of nursing home residents have urinary incontinence. Incontinence may also be related to an underlying medical condition, treatment, or injury.

Incontinence is costly. Every year, Americans spend about $19.5 billion coping with urinary incontinence, and an additional $12.6 billion on urinary urgency and frequency. Of that total, most goes toward managing symptoms or complications rather than toward diagnosis and treatment of the underlying condition. If you are coping with incontinence, you understand all too well the high cost of pads and special absorbent clothing. Add to this the cost of treatment, lost work time, and the emotional toll this condition exacts, and the price is high indeed.

Anatomy of urinary continence

The job of your urinary system is to remove waste products from your blood and help maintain the proper balance of salts and water in your body. The kidneys and ureters constitute the upper urinary tract, and the bladder and urethra make up the lower urinary tract (see Figures 2 and 3, on pages 3 and 4, respectively). Your kidneys filter your blood and create urine to carry away the waste. Urine is a mixture of water, salts, and urea (a waste product produced from protein metabolism). It leaves the kidneys via the ureters, the muscular tubes that deliver urine to the bladder in small amounts.

The bladder. Your bladder is the storage tank that holds urine and allows its release at the appropriate time. In the wall of this balloon-like organ is a layer of smooth muscle, called the detrusor muscle, which enables the bladder to expand and store the liquid until urination. A woman's bladder lies in front of the vagina and uterus (where its ability to expand is noticeably lessened during pregnancy, as the uterus enlarges). A man's bladder is located below his abdomen, between the pubic bone and the rectum.

Figure 1: Men vs. women: Urinary incontinence

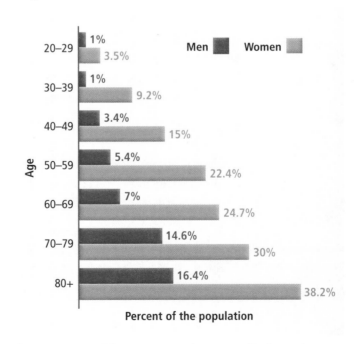

At every age over 20, more women than men suffer from urinary incontinence. This graph shows the percentages of men and women living independently who have moderate or severe problems.

Source: Courtesy Alayne D. Markland, D.O., using data from National Health and Nutrition Examination Surveys 2005–6, 2007–8, and 2009–10.

The urethra. Leading from the bladder to the outside of the body is the urethra, a slim and flexible tube surrounded by smooth muscle. At the junction where the bladder meets the urethra (called the bladder neck), two sets of muscles help hold urine in. The internal urethral sphincter is made up of involuntary muscles that keep a constant pressure on the urethra without conscious effort. The external, or outer, sphincter muscles are under voluntary control. This area is also supported by connective tissue.

In women, the urethra is only about an inch and a half long. Estrogen-sensitive cells line the urethra, producing secretions that help create a tight seal. In men, the urethra is about eight inches long, extending from between the scrotum and rectum to the tip of the penis. Near the bladder, a man's urethra passes through his prostate gland. The prostate, normally the size of a walnut, helps to support the urethra and helps with continence, but it can also create problems if it enlarges or requires removal or other surgery.

Urinary support. The urinary system and the reproductive organs are supported by ligaments and the pelvic floor. The pelvic floor is an important network of muscles and connective tissue that extends from your pubic bone to your tailbone, with openings for the urethra and anus, as well as for the vagina in women. Most of the time, certain pelvic muscles stay contracted to hold the pelvic organs in place against the pull of gravity.

When you are active or trying to avoid urination, you can voluntarily tighten these muscles, along with the external urethral sphincter, to provide added support and prevent leakage. When

Figure 2: Female urinary function

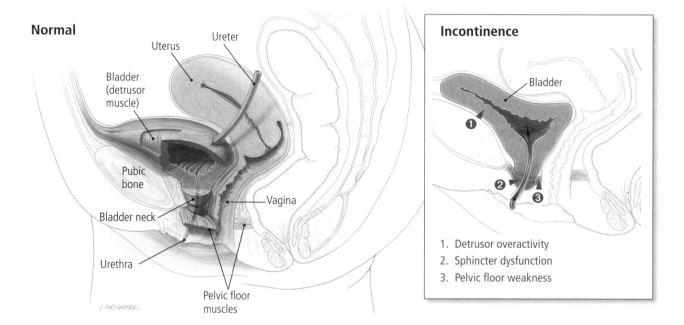

Normal

Uterus
Ureter
Bladder (detrusor muscle)
Pubic bone
Vagina
Bladder neck
Urethra
Pelvic floor muscles

Incontinence

Bladder

❶
❷
❸

1. Detrusor overactivity
2. Sphincter dysfunction
3. Pelvic floor weakness

The bladder's first job is to store urine that has been filtered by the kidneys and delivered through the ureters. Regular stimulation from the sacral nerves keeps the bladder from contracting until you are ready to urinate. Once the bladder is nearly full, a nerve signal is sent to the brain, which releases the brakes on the bladder muscle (detrusor) so it can contract and push the urine out as you voluntarily open your sphincter muscle. In women, incontinence typically results from one of three main problems:

1. The bladder's detrusor muscle can become unstable or overactive, which can cause urge incontinence (also known as overactive bladder).

2. The urinary sphincter that normally opens and closes at your command may weaken, leading to stress incontinence.

3. The pelvic floor muscles may weaken, which can also cause stress incontinence.

you urinate, your pelvic floor muscles and urethral sphincter relax, and your bladder muscles contract, sending the urine from the bladder, through the urethra, and out of the body. When the bladder is empty, the bladder muscles relax, and the sphincter and pelvic muscles tighten.

Urinary nerves. The nervous system helps control urination. Before toilet training, a simple reflex controls the timing of urination. Stretch-detecting sensory nerves in the detrusor muscle signal the spinal cord that the bladder is filling with urine. In response, motor nerves from the spine signal the bladder muscles to contract and the urethra and pelvic floor muscles to relax, allowing urination.

As the brain matures, it is able to override the spinal nerves' automatic signal for the bladder to empty. The bladder gradually becomes capable of storing greater amounts of urine, and a child learns to urinate when it is convenient and socially acceptable. Problems can develop later in life, however.

Types of urinary incontinence

Many things can go wrong with the complex system that allows us to control urination. Incontinence is categorized by the type of problem and, to a lesser extent, by differences in symptoms.

Stress incontinence

If urine leaks out when you jump, cough, or laugh, you may have stress incontinence. Any physical exertion that increases abdominal pressure also puts pressure on the bladder. The word "stress" refers to the physical strain associated with leakage. It has nothing to do with emotion.

Often only a small amount of urine leaks out. In more severe cases, the pressure of a full bladder overcomes the body's ability to hold in urine. The leakage occurs even though the bladder muscles are not contracting and you don't feel the urge to urinate.

Stress incontinence develops when the urethral sphincter, the pelvic floor muscles, or both these

---

Figure 3: Male urinary function

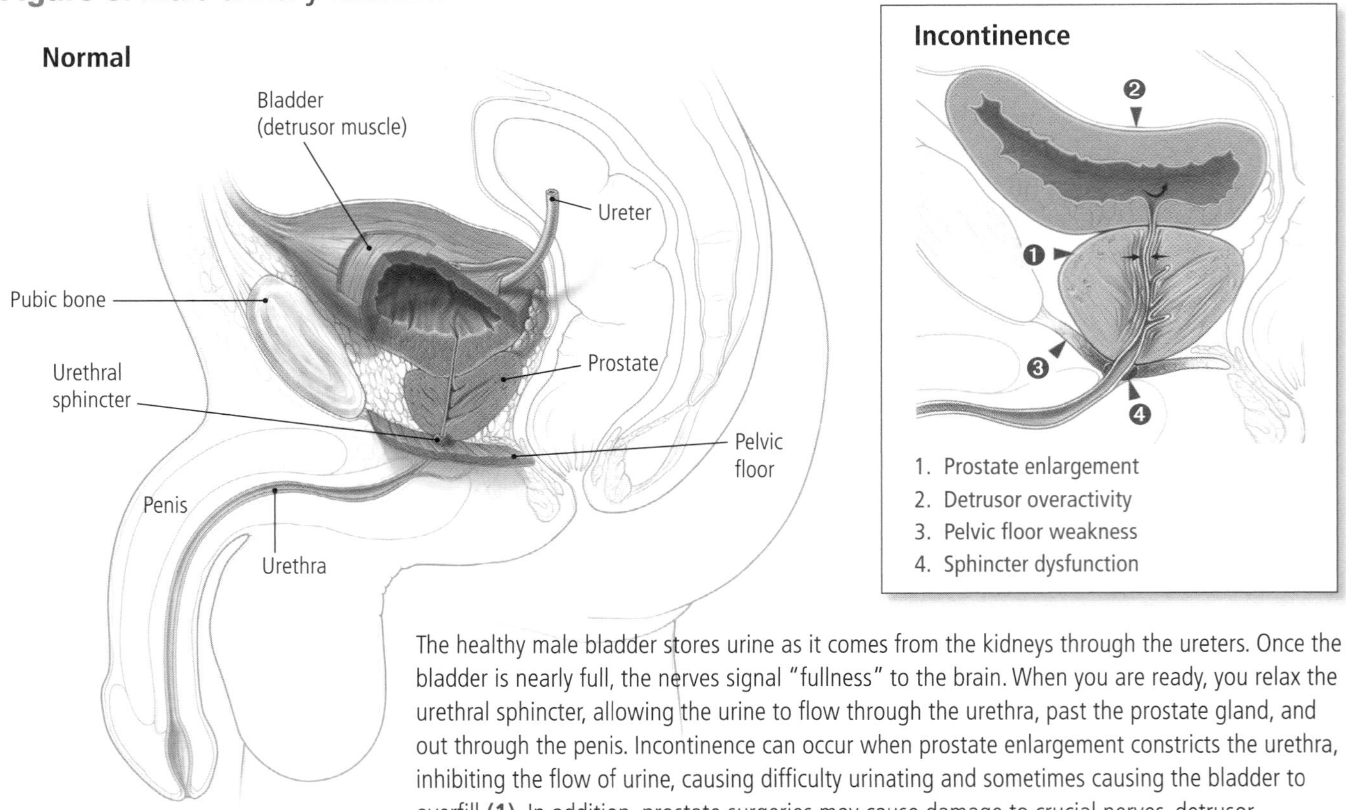

Normal

- Bladder (detrusor muscle)
- Ureter
- Pubic bone
- Prostate
- Urethral sphincter
- Pelvic floor
- Penis
- Urethra

Incontinence

1. Prostate enlargement
2. Detrusor overactivity
3. Pelvic floor weakness
4. Sphincter dysfunction

The healthy male bladder stores urine as it comes from the kidneys through the ureters. Once the bladder is nearly full, the nerves signal "fullness" to the brain. When you are ready, you relax the urethral sphincter, allowing the urine to flow through the urethra, past the prostate gland, and out through the penis. Incontinence can occur when prostate enlargement constricts the urethra, inhibiting the flow of urine, causing difficulty urinating and sometimes causing the bladder to overfill (**1**). In addition, prostate surgeries may cause damage to crucial nerves, detrusor overactivity (**2**), weakened pelvic floor muscles (**3**), or sphincter dysfunction (**4**).

The childbirth connection

It's a little-known fact that many childbirth classes fail to adequately cover: an estimated 40% of women who give birth vaginally go on to develop one or more of the problems collectively known as pelvic floor disorders. These include stress incontinence, overactive bladder, uterine prolapse (in which the uterus drops out of its normal position), anterior vaginal prolapse (also called cystocele, in which the bladder bulges through a weakened vaginal wall), posterior vaginal prolapse (also called rectocele, in which the rectum bulges through a weakened vaginal wall), and fecal incontinence. Both cystocele and rectocele can be thought of as types of hernias. These disorders often grow worse over time, and one out of 10 women eventually undergoes a surgical repair.

Vaginal delivery can lead to pelvic floor damage as the baby stretches the pelvic floor muscles and other tissues on its way through the birth canal, sometimes causing tearing or other damage. Research shows that a number of factors raise the risk of damage for women who deliver vaginally, including these:

- older age of the mother
- greater weight of the baby
- higher number of vaginal births
- longer second stage of labor (the pushing stage)
- vaginal delivery assisted by forceps or a vacuum device
- episiotomy (a surgical cut made to expand the vaginal opening during vaginal delivery).

What are the solutions?

Delivery by cesarean section sometimes protects against severe incontinence. However, the difference in urinary incontinence rates following cesarean versus vaginal delivery tends to diminish within a few years of giving birth. For example, a 2013 study found that the same percentage of women had incontinence two years after delivering their first baby, whether vaginally or by elective cesarean section.

A review from Norway evaluated the benefit of various strategies for avoiding incontinence after childbirth. Women were less likely to experience incontinence after childbirth if they were nonsmokers, were of normal weight before pregnancy and returned to that weight afterward, did not experience constipation during or after pregnancy, and performed pelvic muscle exercises during and after pregnancy.

The use of episiotomy during childbirth has declined steadily, but millions of women have had episiotomies in the past. It was previously believed that an episiotomy helped prevent tearing of the vagina and damage to the pelvic floor. However, evidence has failed to confirm any benefit. And an episiotomy may cause more damage than it prevents. For example, studies in the journal *Obstetrics and Gynecology* found that women who had an episiotomy during their first or subsequent deliveries were more likely to experience tears in the anal sphincter. After sphincter tear and repair, about half of women experience fecal or gas incontinence. For many women, the symptoms improve or disappear within a few months, but others sustain persistent or worsening problems, or find that symptoms reappear after subsequent deliveries.

Besides episiotomy, other major factors contributing to sphincter tears were larger babies, a prolonged second stage of labor, and forceps delivery. Vacuum delivery had a smaller risk of sphincter tear than forceps delivery. Gentle delivery techniques and slow, gradual induction (when induction is necessary) would go a long way toward sparing women incontinence resulting from childbirth. For example, the Norwegian review found good evidence that using warm packs on the perineum (the tissue between the anus and vulva) during delivery can reduce the risk of later incontinence.

structures have been weakened or damaged and cannot dependably hold in urine. Stress incontinence is divided into two subtypes.

- In urethral hypermobility, the bladder and urethra shift downward when abdominal pressure rises, and there is no hammock-like support for the urethra to be compressed against to keep it closed.
- In urethral incompetence (formerly called intrinsic sphincter deficiency), problems in the urinary sphincter keep it from closing fully or allow it to pop open under pressure.

Many experts believe that women who have delivered a baby vaginally are more likely to develop stress incontinence because giving birth has stretched and possibly damaged the urethral sphincter muscles and nerves. Generally, the larger the baby, the longer the labor, the older the mother, and the greater the number of births, the more likely that incontinence will result (see "The childbirth connection," above).

Age is likewise a factor in stress incontinence. As a woman gets older, the muscles in her pelvic floor and urethra weaken, and it takes less pressure for the urethra to open and allow leakage. Declining estrogen can also play some role, although it is not clear how much. Many women do not experience symptoms until after menopause.

In men, the most frequent cause of stress incontinence is urinary sphincter damage sustained through prostate surgery or a pelvic fracture.

Lung conditions that cause frequent coughing, such as emphysema and cystic fibrosis, can also contribute to stress incontinence in both men and women.

Overactive bladder (urge incontinence)

If you feel a strong urge to urinate even when your bladder isn't full, your incontinence might be related to overactive bladder, sometimes called urge incontinence or urgency incontinence. This condition occurs in both men and women and involves an overwhelming urge to urinate immediately, frequently followed by loss of urine before you can reach a bathroom (see "Key-in-the-door syndrome," above right). Even if you never have an accident, urgency and urinary frequency can interfere with your work and social life because of the need to keep running to the bathroom.

Urgency occurs when the bladder muscle, the detrusor, begins to contract and signals a need to urinate, which can happen even when the bladder is not full. Another name for this phenomenon is detrusor overactivity.

Overactive bladder can result from physical problems that keep your body from halting involuntary bladder muscle contractions. Such problems include damage to the brain, the spine, or the nerves extending from the spine to the bladder—for example, from an accident, diabetes, or neurological disease. Irritating substances within the bladder, such as those produced during an infection, might also cause the bladder muscle to contract.

Most often there is no identifiable cause for overactive bladder, but people are more likely to develop the problem as they age. Postmenopausal women, in particular, tend to develop this condition, perhaps because of age-related changes in the bladder lining and muscle. African American women with incontinence are more likely to report symptoms of overactive bladder than stress incontinence, while the reverse is true in white women.

A condition called myofascial pelvic pain syndrome has been identified with symptoms that include overactive bladder accompanied by pain in the pelvic

> ## ▶ Key-in-the-door syndrome
>
> Do you get an overwhelming urge to urinate just when you arrive home and start to open the door? Also called "latchkey incontinence," this phenomenon is a good demonstration of the bladder-brain connection. When you feel the urge to urinate as you're going home, you suppress it until you arrive. Eventually, the bladder becomes conditioned to associate arriving home with urinating, and the urge comes on whether or not your bladder is full. This is not a "psychological" problem, but a reflex-conditioning problem, much as when you salivate upon smelling something good to eat.

area or a sense of aching, heaviness, or burning.

In addition, infections of the urinary tract, bladder, or prostate can cause temporary urgency. Partial blockage of the urinary tract by a bladder stone, a tumor (rarely), or, in men, an enlarged prostate (a condition known as benign prostatic hyperplasia, or BPH) can cause urgency, frequency, and sometimes urge incontinence. Surgery for prostate cancer or BPH can trigger symptoms of overactive bladder, as can freezing (cryotherapy) and radiation seed treatment (brachytherapy) for prostate cancer.

Neurological diseases (such as Parkinson's disease and multiple sclerosis) can also result in urge incontinence, as can a stroke. Three months after being discharged from the hospital following a stroke, about 44% of patients have incontinence; by one year later, 38% do.

Mixed incontinence

If you have symptoms of both overactive bladder and stress incontinence, you likely have mixed incontinence, a combination of both types. Most women with incontinence have both stress and urge symptoms—a challenging situation. Mixed incontinence also occurs in men who have had prostate removal or surgery for an enlarged prostate, and in frail older people of either sex.

Overflow incontinence

If your bladder never empties adequately, you might experience urine leakage, with or without feeling a need to go. Overflow incontinence occurs when something blocks urine from flowing normally out of the bladder, as in the case of prostate enlargement that partially closes off the urethra. It can also occur in both men and women if the bladder muscle (detrusor) becomes underactive (the opposite of an overactive bladder). When that happens, you don't feel an urge to urinate, and the bladder is unable to push out most of the urine. Eventually the bladder becomes overfilled, or distended, and the urine leaks out. The bladder might also spasm at random times, causing leakage. This condition is sometimes related to diabetes or cardiovascular disease.

Men are much more frequently diagnosed with overflow incontinence than women because it is often caused by prostate-related conditions. In addition to enlarged prostate, other possible causes of urine blockage include tumors, bladder stones, or scar tissue. If a woman has severe prolapse of her uterus or bladder (meaning that the organ has dropped out of its proper position), her urethra can become kinked like a bent garden hose, interfering with the flow of urine. This can also happen if a woman has had surgery for stress incontinence.

Nerve damage (from injuries, childbirth, past surgeries, radiation treatment, or diseases such as diabetes, multiple sclerosis, or shingles) and aging often prevent the bladder muscle from contracting normally. Medications that prevent bladder muscle contraction or that make you unaware of the urge to urinate can also result in overflow incontinence.

Functional incontinence

If your urinary tract is functioning properly but other illnesses or disabilities are preventing you from staying dry, you might have what is known as functional incontinence. For example, if an illness rendered you unaware or unconcerned about the need to find a toilet, you would become incontinent. Medications, dementia, or mental illness can decrease awareness of the need to find a toilet.

Even if your urinary system is fine, it can be extremely hard for you to avoid accidents if you have trouble getting to a toilet. This problem can affect anyone with a condition that makes it excessively difficult to move to the bathroom and undress in time. This includes problems as diverse as having arthritis, being hospitalized or restrained, or being too far away from a toilet.

If a medication (such as a diuretic used to treat high blood pressure or heart failure) causes you to produce abnormally large amounts of urine, you could develop incontinence that requires a change in treatment, such as taking your diuretic earlier in the day to avoid getting up at night to urinate. If you make most of your urine at night, the result might be nocturnal (nighttime) enuresis, or bedwetting.

Reflex incontinence

Reflex incontinence occurs when the bladder muscle contracts and urine leaks (often in large amounts) without any warning or urge. This can happen as a result of damage to the nerves that normally warn the brain that the bladder is filling. Reflex incontinence usually appears in people with serious neurological impairment from multiple sclerosis, spinal cord injury, other injuries, or damage from surgery or radiation treatment. ⬇

Evaluating urinary incontinence

Many people never tell a physician that they are incontinent, and that leads to prolonged and largely needless suffering. In 70% of cases, incontinence can be cured or significantly improved. The treatment of incontinence has advanced greatly and is changing all the time, so don't be reluctant to seek help now, even if previous attempts brought you little relief.

If you are comfortable with your primary care physician, start there. If your symptoms seem to be connected with a specific medical event, such as childbirth, surgery, or starting a new prescription, the physician involved in that treatment might be your first choice. A man who has had prostate symptoms or treatment may choose to consult a urologist. A woman may choose to see a urologist who has been trained to treat bladder control problems or a urogynecologist—a gynecologist with board-certified special training in incontinence (also known as a female pelvic medicine and reconstructive surgery specialist). Physicians vary widely in their training and interest in incontinence. If a doctor seems uncomfortable or uninformed discussing the subject, presents limited options, or seems unduly pessimistic about your condition, seek another opinion.

To pinpoint and treat the underlying problem, your physician will need you to describe your symptoms in as much detail as possible. You might be asked to keep a diary of urination, leakage, and fluid intake for a few days (see "Keeping a bladder diary," page 15). At your visit, be prepared to give a full medical history, including details on all surgeries, pregnancies, and any medications you are taking, since certain drugs can cause incontinence by increasing urine production or relaxing muscles of the bladder or urethra (see Table 1, below). You may also need to answer specific questions such as these:

- When did the incontinence start?
- How often do you have leakage?
- Is it worse during the day or night?
- What brings it on? Do you have any warning?
- What makes it worse?
- Does anything make it better?

Table 1: Medications that can cause urinary incontinence

MEDICATION	EFFECT	SYMPTOMS
Diuretics, such as hydrochlorothiazide (Esidrix, Hydrodiuril, Oretic), furosemide (Lasix), bumetanide (Bumex), triamterene with hydrochlorothiazide (Maxzide)	Increase urine production by the kidney.	Frequent urination, overactive bladder, urgency, and stress incontinence.
Muscle relaxants and sedatives, such as diazepam (Valium), chlordiazepoxide (Librium), lorazepam (Ativan)	Cause sedation or drowsiness; relax urethra.	Frequent urination, stress incontinence, lack of concern or desire to use the toilet.
Narcotics, such as oxycodone (Percocet), meperidine (Demerol), morphine	Cause sedation or drowsiness; relax bladder, causing retention of urine.	Lack of concern or desire to use the toilet, difficulty in starting urinary stream, straining to void, voiding with a weak stream, leaking between urinations, frequency incontinence.
Antihistamines, such as diphenhydramine (Benadryl) and chlorpheniramine (Chlor-Trimeton)	Relax bladder, causing retention of urine.	Overflow incontinence.
Alpha-adrenergic antagonists, such as terazosin (Hytrin), doxazosin (Cardura)	Relax the bladder outlet muscle.	Leaking when coughing, sneezing, laughing, exercising, etc.

- Do you generally leak a little (damp underwear), a moderate amount (your underwear is soaked), or a lot (your clothing gets soaked and all the urine in your bladder comes out)?
- Do you leak urine during intercourse or with orgasm?
- How much do you drink on a typical day (including water, soda, juice, caffeinated and alcoholic beverages, and other fluids)?
- How often do you go to the toilet to empty your bladder during the daytime? How often when you are trying to sleep?
- Do you have other problems urinating? After you urinate, does your bladder still feel full? Do you have trouble starting the urine flow? Is the stream weak or strong? Is urination ever painful?
- Have you also had trouble controlling your bowel movements?
- Are you using pads or other means to manage your incontinence? How is it working? Have you altered your activities because of incontinence?

The physical exam

For this exam, your clinician places more focus on your nervous system, abdomen, and genital area than during a standard physical. The clinician checks your reflexes, assesses your muscle strength, and observes whether you can distinguish the touch of something sharp from something dull. To test nerves in the genital area, the doctor may stroke the skin near your anus and watch for a normal muscle contraction. In women, the doctor gently taps the clitoris and looks for a subtle muscle contraction of the anus, which is a normal reflex.

None of these tests is painful or uncomfortable. If the doctor observes problems with any functions that rely on the same nerves as those that control urinary continence, it can mean that these nerves are involved in your bladder symptoms.

During the abdominal exam, the doctor presses on your abdomen to feel your bladder and check other areas for hernias, tenderness, or any signs of tumor, infection, scarring from previous surgeries, or an impacted bowel.

▶ Is it cancer?

Incontinence can be a symptom of bladder cancer, but it is rarely the first or only sign of this disease. If you have other symptoms, such as blood in your urine, your physician is likely to suggest specific tests to rule out bladder cancer. Bladder cancer is much less common than cancers of the breast, colon, lung, or prostate.

Both men and women provide a urine sample, which is checked immediately for blood, sugar, or large amounts of bacteria (normal urine is sterile). Blood can indicate irritation of the urinary tract. If there is such irritation, the cause must be determined. If sugar is detected, your physician might suspect diabetes, which can increase your urine volume and make incontinence more likely. Bacteria indicate possible infection. As a more specific test, a urine sample may be sent to a laboratory to be cultured; if harmful bacteria are detected, a sensitivity test can identify the appropriate antibiotic to treat the infection.

For women. During a thorough pelvic exam, the clinician inserts a gloved finger into the vagina to help assess the strength of the pelvic floor muscles and to see whether the bladder or uterus has prolapsed (dropped out of normal position). If you hear the term POP, it may mean your clinician is using the Pelvic Organ Prolapse Quantification system, also called the POP-Q system, as a way of measuring and grading the degree of prolapse of the pelvic organs to help guide decisions about treatment.

The clinician might ask you to contract your muscles as if you were trying to avoid urinating or passing gas, or to cough during the exam to see if urine spurts out of the urethra. The clinician might repeat the exam while you are standing up.

With a speculum in place, the clinician observes whether the tissue lining your vagina is dry or shows other signs that it lacks estrogen. That would indicate that your urethral lining (not visible during the exam) is likely to show a similar lack of this hormone. The clinician may insert a cotton swab coated with numbing jelly (such as Xylocaine) into your urethra just up into the bladder to observe how the angle of the swab changes when you bear down as if trying to have a bowel movement. A large change indicates poor support of the urethra and points toward a diagnosis of stress incontinence.

The clinician might also look for direct evidence of stress incontinence. You may be asked to stand with one leg up on a stool, holding a paper towel over your crotch; if urine appears on the paper towel after you cough, that's a positive stress test. This test is usually performed at the beginning of your physical, when you have a full bladder. Afterward, you can urinate to increase your comfort during the rest of the exam.

Occasionally, if stress incontinence is suspected but is not observed during the exam, the clinician may give you a preweighed pad to wear while doing a series of exercises. The pad is then weighed again to determine how much leakage has occurred. You might go home with a package of pads to wear and save in sealed plastic bags over a 24-hour period, so that total leakage can be estimated. This is often called the "pad test."

For men. The doctor examines the penis for signs of constriction of the foreskin or an abnormal narrowing, or stenosis, of the urethra, which can result from scarring or infection. The doctor conducts a digital rectal exam, which involves inserting a gloved finger into the rectum to feel the size and texture of the prostate gland and assess the strength of the pelvic muscles. You may be asked to contract your muscles as if you were trying to avoid urinating or passing gas.

Urodynamic testing

If your condition is not easily diagnosed by a physical exam and a discussion of your symptoms, or if previous treatments have not improved your symptoms of incontinence, your doctor may suggest urodynamic testing, a series of specialized tests that help evaluate your urinary system in action. Many doctors who diagnose patients with urinary problems have a urodynamic testing lab outfitted with a special chair and computer equipment that can help obtain measurements of urinary pressure and flow (see Figure 4, below left).

Urodynamic testing is available for both men and women. For women, the testing may be done by a nurse, technician, or physician. Often the physician is a urologist or a gynecologist who is board certified in female pelvic medicine and reconstructive surgery. Men should consult a urologist, another type of board-certified specialist.

The usefulness of urodynamic testing depends on the experience of the tester, the choice of tests, and the type of incontinence. For example, urodynamic tests are very sensitive in detecting stress incontinence, but asking patients about their symptoms is almost as good, and is even more effective when supplemented with a bladder diary (see "Keeping a bladder diary," page 15).

Urodynamic testing will likely be recommended if your symptoms point toward more than one type of incontinence, if you have had previous surgery on your bladder or sphincters, if surgery is planned, or if you do not improve after standard treatments.

Your urodynamic test is likely to include one or more of the following procedures.

Uroflowmetry

For this test, you start with a full bladder and urinate into a funnel at a special urinal or commode that auto-

---

Figure 4: Detecting bladder problems

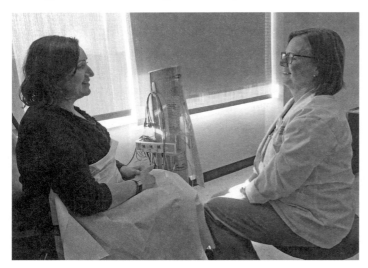

Before you begin urodynamic testing, your doctor will ask you to describe your symptoms and your personal health history. Once you are in the urodynamic testing lab (above), you'll sit in a specially designed chair equipped with sensitive catheters that feed information from your bladder to a computer that records bladder volume, pressure, rate of flow, and leakage.

Photo courtesy of May M. Wakamatsu, M.D.

Finding a clinician

To get help for incontinence, your primary care physician is a good place to start. But not all physicians have the necessary interest or experience. If your doctor seems unable to help, keep looking. There are several kinds of health professionals and several types of clinics that work with people with these conditions. For contact information for the organizations named here, see "Resources," page 47.

Urogynecologists. These are gynecologists who have taken additional training in problems affecting a woman's bladder and pelvis—including urinary and fecal incontinence or prolapse. Check your state's listing on the American Urogynecologic Society website. This board-certified subspecialty is also known as female pelvic medicine and reconstructive surgery.

Urologists. These medical doctors treat the urinary systems of both men and women as well as the male reproductive organs. The American Urological Association website has a physician locator.

Gastroenterologists and colorectal surgeons. These doctors have training in treating conditions of the gastrointestinal tract, including fecal incontinence. If you have diarrhea or digestive symptoms in addition to incontinence, start with a gastroenterologist, particularly if there is no known childbirth injury or other trauma to the sphincter. Several organizations offer physician locators. Again, keep in mind that not all gastroenterologists have given this problem much attention. A colorectal surgeon should be prepared to offer you a range of surgical and nonsurgical options for treatment. The American Society of Colon and Rectal Surgeons has a directory of members.

Biofeedback professionals. Health professionals who practice this technique include nurses and physical or occupational therapists. Look for someone with experience in bowel or bladder training. Start by asking the physician treating your incontinence, or contact the Biofeedback Certification International Alliance.

Pelvic floor physical therapists. If you need help learning to strengthen and control your pelvic floor muscles and to use other behavioral strategies to maintain continence, a growing number of physical therapists specialize in this area and have undergone advanced training to earn a Certificate of Achievement of Pelvic Physical Therapy. Ask your physician for a referral, or contact the American Physical Therapy Association.

Nurse specialists. If you are having skin problems related to incontinence or if you have not been able to find acceptable ways to manage your incontinence, a specialist in continence or ostomy nursing can offer practical advice. Contact the Wound, Ostomy, and Continence Nurses Society.

You can find teams that include many of the clinicians listed above at specialized centers, such as these:

Anorectal physiology labs. Run by clinicians and equipped to evaluate fecal incontinence, these facilities are often located in hospital departments specializing in motility disorders or functional bowel disorders (most likely gastroenterology, surgery, or urogynecology departments) as well as in some private practices.

Pelvic floor disorder centers. Some hospitals have developed clinics to provide one-stop shopping for the evaluation and treatment of many pelvic floor disorders, including urinary and fecal incontinence. These clinics may combine the expertise of many specialists, including urogynecologists, colorectal surgeons, urologists, gastroenterologists, neurologists, physiatrists (physicians who deal with muscle and skeletal problems and rehabilitation), and physical therapists.

---

matically measures the amount you produce and the rate of the flow. A slow flow might indicate an obstruction in the urethra or a weak bladder muscle. This test is quick and noninvasive.

Post-void residual volume

This test measures the amount of urine left in your bladder after you urinate. Two techniques are used to measure this. The physician may insert a flexible tube (called a catheter) through your urethra into the bladder to draw off the remaining fluid (which also provides an uncontaminated sample for urine culture and prepares you for further tests). Being catheterized usually causes only mild discomfort. Alternatively,

the amount of urine in your bladder can be visualized using a specialized ultrasound machine called a bladder scanner. This is quicker and more comfortable, and it avoids the possibility that inserting a catheter could cause an infection or traumatize the lining of the urethra. However, it can be less accurate.

Measuring residual urine volume is particularly valuable if you are troubled by repeated urinary tract infections, if you have a neurological disorder, or if your doctor suspects that a blockage is preventing your bladder from emptying properly.

Cystometry

This test monitors how the pressure builds up in your

bladder as it fills with urine, how much urine your bladder can hold, and at what point you feel the urge to urinate (see Figure 5, below).

During cystometry, a very narrow catheter is placed in your bladder to measure pressure. Through the catheter, the technician slowly fills your bladder with sterile water. The catheter measures the pressure inside your bladder and inside the urethra; an additional small pressure catheter may also be inserted into your rectum (for men) or vaginal canal (for women). You tell the physician when you first feel the urge to urinate, when the urge becomes strong, and other sensations (pain, temperature changes, and the symptoms that brought you to the doctor).

This test detects abnormal contractions or spasms of your detrusor muscle during filling, indicating incontinence caused by an overactive bladder (either alone or along with stress incontinence). At several points during the filling, you may be asked to cough or bear down so the doctor can see whether fluid comes out of the urethra. This measurement is sometimes called leak point pressure.

A low leak point pressure is a sign of stress incontinence. If it is extremely low (you start to leak as soon as you begin bearing down), it may mean that age-related changes or scar tissue is preventing your urethra from closing well enough to prevent urine leakage, resulting in the type of stress incontinence called urethral incompetence.

Once your bladder is filled to the point where you have a strong urge, you will urinate, and the pressure and volume are measured. By monitoring pressure while you urinate, this test can distinguish whether a low flow is due to weak bladder contractions or something blocking the flow. Portions of the test may be repeated while you are standing, which makes stress incontinence more apparent.

In women, urogynecologists often perform a test called a urethral pressure profile. The bladder/urethral catheter is drawn through the urethra very slowly, and

Figure 5: Pressure test (cystometry)

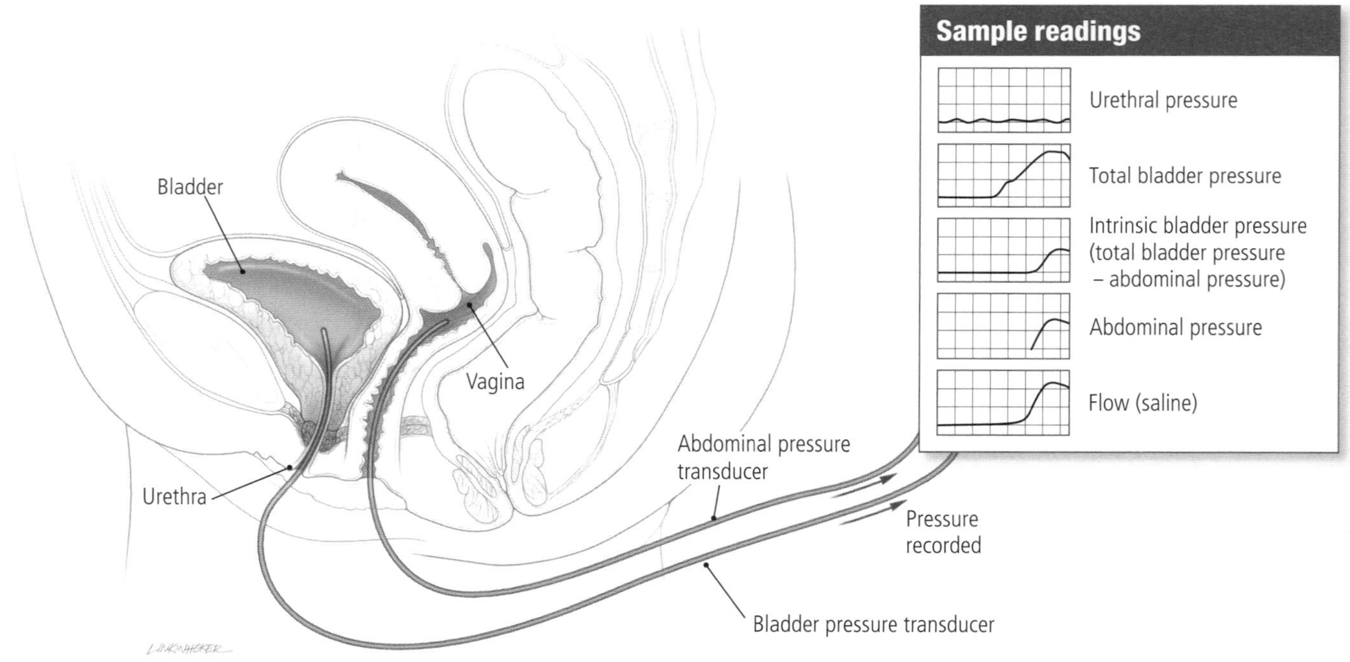

For men or women, a cystometry test measures the pressure in the bladder, urethra, and abdomen. A catheter in the bladder fills the bladder with fluid and measures pressure in centimeters of water. Another catheter, placed in the vagina for women or the rectum for men, reflects the pressure in the abdomen. Cystometry can reveal detrusor overactivity, stress incontinence from sphincter weakness, or weak pelvic floor muscles.

the urethral pressure is measured. If the pressure is low, that indicates your urethral sphincter is weak, a cause of stress incontinence.

Electromyography (EMG)

In this test, small electrode patches are placed in the crotch area to pick up electrical current that is created when the pelvic floor muscles contract. Called a surface EMG, this test may help determine whether the activities of the bladder and urethra are coordinated with each other.

If your doctor suspects that the nerves to your urinary sphincter are seriously damaged, or that the sphincter muscle is responding inappropriately to nerve signals, he or she may insert a thin needle electrode into the muscle of the urethra to perform a more accurate EMG. This test may also be performed by a neurologist.

Because most people find that the EMG causes some pain, it is not done routinely.

Cystography

A cystogram, or voiding cystourethrogram, is an x-ray test. The test itself may be performed during cystometry or uroflowmetry, or both, but a fluid visible on x-ray is substituted for the sterile water. At various points in the process, x-rays are taken as you cough or bear down and as you urinate. This test can pinpoint the location of a blockage or reveal an abnormally open urethra.

Video-urodynamic study

Using highly specialized equipment, this technique combines cystometry, uroflowmetry, and cystography into a single computerized test. This equipment can simultaneously measure urine flow and pressure in the bladder and rectum. The test may provide useful information about your bladder and urethral function, especially if you have problems voiding (such as being able to begin urinating only in a certain position). The equipment for video-urodynamic testing is expensive and not widely used.

Other evaluation procedures

Depending on your symptoms, other tests may be performed at the same visit as your urodynamic testing.

Cystoscopy

Using a lighted telescope at the end of a thin tube called a cystoscope, your doctor can inspect the inside of your urethra and bladder for signs of infection, abnormal growths, bladder stones, scarring, or mesh or stitches from previous surgeries. This test is used in both men and women, but it is easier for women to undergo comfortably because the urethra is shorter.

For the test, you lie on your back. A numbing jelly is placed into your urethra, and the cystoscope is inserted until the end is inside your bladder. Sterile water is passed through the thin tube to fill your bladder and optimize the picture. You may feel some discomfort and the need to urinate when your bladder is filled. After about two to three minutes, the cystoscope is removed, and you can use the toilet.

Ultrasound

Ultrasound uses sound waves rather than x-rays to create an image of internal organs. You may undergo an abdominal or transvaginal ultrasound exam to look at the structure and position of your kidneys, bladder, and prostate; to visualize leakage in stress incontinence; to detect abnormalities such as tumors, kidney stones, or fibroids; or to evaluate treatment with bulking agents (see "Bulking agents for stress incontinence," page 24). An ultrasound exam takes about half an hour and is painless. ♥

Treating urinary incontinence

Treatment choices for urinary incontinence range from lifestyle changes to surgery. Your treatment will depend on the underlying problems causing the incontinence. But keep in mind that no treatment works perfectly, and you may have to try more than one approach before you find the one that best suits your needs (see "Quick guide: What to do for urinary incontinence," below right). Treatments may be different for men and women. Because there are a variety of options, your preferences are important in developing a plan.

It's also important to know that less invasive treatments, such as biofeedback or pelvic floor exercises, are a good first step and can be helpful, but may not be as effective as some surgical procedures. To make the most of these approaches, ask your doctor about a referral to a physical therapist specializing in pelvic floor disorders. If he or she can't suggest a local practitioner, both men and woman can find a therapist with experience treating incontinence by going to the American Physical Therapy Association's online locator (see "Resources," page 47).

If you do need surgery, the good news is that procedures are becoming less invasive and require shorter recovery times. You and your physician need to decide which approach is most appropriate for you. Check with your health plan to find out which therapies are covered.

Treatment for urinary incontinence is an area of active research, and new approaches are under development.

Bladder training

You might be teaching your bladder some bad habits—habits that can gradually result in incontinence or frequent bathroom breaks. For example, if you rou-

---

Quick guide: What to do for urinary incontinence

Use this guide to help pinpoint the strategies that may work for your type of urinary incontinence. Then consult the appropriate section in this chapter to read more.

Stress incontinence

Lifestyle changes
- Fluid management (page 16)

Muscle conditioning
- Pelvic floor physical therapy (page 18)
- Biofeedback (page 18)
- Electrical stimulation (page 19)

Surgical procedures
- Sling (page 25)
- Bladder neck suspension (page 27)
- Artificial urinary sphincter (page 28)

Other procedures
- Injection of bulking agents (page 24)

Overactive bladder

Lifestyle changes
- Bladder training (page 14)
- Decrease or eliminate caffeine
- Fluid management (page 16)

Muscle conditioning
- Pelvic floor physical therapy (page 18)
- Biofeedback (page 18)
- Electrical stimulation (page 19)

Medications
- Anticholinergics (page 21)
- Antidepressants (tricyclic; page 21)

- Beta-3 adrenergic agonist (page 22)
- Estrogen (page 22)

Surgical procedures
- Sacral nerve stimulation (severe overactive bladder in men, or overactive bladder in women; page 22)

Other procedures
- Injection of botulinum toxin (page 23)
- Percutaneous tibial nerve stimulation (page 23)

Other conditions

Medications
- Alpha-adrenergic antagonists, for overflow incontinence in men (page 21)
- Antidepressants (tricyclic), for nocturia (page 21)
- Antidiuretic hormone, for bedwetting (page 22)
- Cholinergic, for overflow incontinence (page 22)

Surgical procedures
- Artificial urinary sphincter, for reflex incontinence (page 28)
- Sacral nerve stimulation, for overflow incontinence or urinary retention (page 22)

---

tinely urinate before your bladder is full, the bladder learns to signal the need to go when less volume is present. That can set up a vicious cycle, as you respond to the new urges and teach your bladder to cry "run" when less and less urine is present.

Luckily, old bladders can learn new tricks. Bladder training, a program of urinating on a schedule, enables you to gradually increase the amount of urine you can comfortably hold. Bladder training is a mainstay of treatment for urinary frequency and overactive bladder in both women and men, alone or in conjunction with medications or other techniques. It can also help prevent or lessen symptoms of overactive bladder that may emerge after surgery for stress incontinence.

In one study, women ages 55 and older who participated in six weekly bladder training sessions had half as many episodes of leakage compared with a group of women who didn't undergo bladder training.

You can see a health professional for bladder training, or you can try it on your own. Because bladder training is low-cost and low-risk, your clinician may encourage you to try it first, even before specific diagnostic tests are performed. Here's a step-by-step bladder-training technique:

1. Keep track. For a day or two, keep track of the times you urinate or leak urine during the day (see "Keeping a bladder diary," below).

2. Calculate. On average, how many hours do you wait between urinations during the day?

3. Choose an interval. Based on your typical interval between urinations, select a starting interval for training that is 15 minutes longer. If your typical interval is one hour, make your starting interval one hour and 15 minutes.

4. Hold back. When you start training, empty your bladder first thing in the morning and not again until the interval you've set. If the time arrives before you feel the urge, go anyway. If the urge hits first,

Keeping a bladder diary

Complete the information for a 24-hour period, both day and night.

- Begin with your first urination upon getting out of bed in the morning. Record the time and approximate urine output. (Use a measuring cup or a special collection device that fits under the toilet seat.)
- Record all the fluids you drink, including the type of fluid (for example, coffee, juice, water, etc.), the amount in ounces, and the time.
- Continue to record approximate urine output and time at each urination. Note if there was any accidental leakage.

	TRIPS TO THE BATHROOM How much urine did you void?	ACCIDENTAL LEAKING			FLUID INTAKE 1 cup = 8 oz	
Time	Amount voided	Leak 1 = few drops 2 = soaked pad 3 = emptied	What were you doing when you leaked?	Was there an urge before the leak?	What kind	How much
		1　2　3		Yes　No		
		1　2　3		Yes　No		
		1　2　3		Yes　No		
		1　2　3		Yes　No		
		1　2　3		Yes　No		
		1　2　3		Yes　No		
		1　2　3		Yes　No		
		1　2　3		Yes　No		
		1　2　3		Yes　No		

remind yourself that your bladder isn't necessarily full, and use whatever techniques you can to delay going. Try the pelvic floor exercises sometimes called Kegels (see "Pelvic floor exercises," page 17), or simply try to wait another five minutes before walking slowly to the bathroom.

5. Increase your interval. Once you are comfortable with your set interval, increase it by 15 minutes. Over several weeks or months, you may find you are able to wait much longer and that you experience far fewer feelings of urgency or episodes of urge incontinence. After four to eight weeks, if you think you have improved, do another diary. Compare your initial diary to your second diary to note the improvements in voiding intervals and voided volumes—this reinforces the bladder training process. Set a goal of waiting at least three hours between voids.

Fluid management

Do you have a drinking problem? Not just alcohol, but water, soda, coffee, tea, or juice? For some people who drink more fluids than they really need, eliminating excess fluid intake is all it takes to bring incontinence under control. For example, in a British study, reducing fluid intake by 25%—that is, enjoying your usual beverages, but pouring each cup or glass only three-quarters full—significantly reduced overactive bladder symptoms and nocturia (the regular need to urinate more than twice during the night).

To determine whether you're drinking more liquids than you require, review your bladder diary with your physician. If your urine output is much higher than 48 ounces, you may be drinking too much fluid. This isn't necessarily unhealthy, but it forces your bladder to handle more urine and may invite or aggravate incontinence. Cutting back may be helpful.

On the other hand, if your output is much lower than 30 to 40 ounces, you may need to drink more. Insufficient fluid can increase your risk for urinary tract infection and, in some people, create a frequent urge to urinate because the concentrated urine irritates the bladder lining.

To help manage the amount of fluid you're consuming every day and control your symptoms, you can try the following technique. (Note: Do not try this if you engage in strenuous exercise or have a medical condition, such as a propensity toward forming kidney stones, that requires more fluid consumption.)

- Drink only when you feel thirsty, and don't exceed a total of six to eight 8-ounce cups of fluid per day from all sources, including soup or milk in your cereal.
- Don't drink more than 8 ounces at a time. (This could be challenging if you're used to drinking from larger containers, such as 12-ounce cans or 20-ounce bottles of soda.)
- Don't guzzle. The faster your bladder fills, the more likely you are to feel urgency.
- Minimize caffeinated drinks, which act as diuretics.

Debunking a myth: You do not need eight cups of water a day

The old advice to drink at least eight glasses of water a day no longer holds water, so to speak—particularly if you are prone to urinary incontinence. Instead, 48 ounces to 64 ounces a day—six to eight cups—is fine. What's more, that includes all fluids, not just water.

Where did the old recommendation come from? Some experts think it was based on a misunderstanding. It has been traced to the 1940s, when the National Academy of Sciences published a recommended daily intake of 1 milliliter of fluid for each calorie burned—a little over eight cups for a typical 2,000-calorie diet. However, the statement then explained that most of this fluid could be obtained via the liquid contained in foods.

Regardless, the eight-glasses-a-day dictum caught on. Indeed, today people frequently consume much more as they tote giant water bottles, buy super-sized soft drinks, and follow the dictates of programs that promise you can lose weight by drinking as much as a quart of fluid at a time. Other people drink extra water or other liquids as part of a special diet that purports to purify or detoxify the liver or other body organs. But a person with normal liver and kidney function can rest assured that these organs will rid the body of toxins on their own. And drinking water won't help you lose weight unless you are drinking it to replace high-calorie drinks you might ordinarily consume, such as soda and fruit juice.

- Minimize carbonated drinks, which can irritate sensitive bladders.
- Decrease or eliminate your consumption of alcohol, which acts as a diuretic.
- If you are thirsty because it is hot or you have exercised, don't hesitate to drink water.

Pelvic floor exercises

Another approach for men and women who want to try nonsurgical methods first is to strengthen the muscles of the pelvic floor through exercise. The strength and proper action of your pelvic floor muscles are important in maintaining continence. Like weakened or damaged muscles elsewhere in your body, they can usually be strengthened with regular exercise and, if needed, physical therapy.

It may seem odd, but overly tight pelvic floor muscles, too, can cause incontinence. That's because tight muscles (resulting from pelvic, back, or hip surgery or other causes) can't relax when they are supposed to. Then, when the time comes for them to contract to control the flow of urine, they can't, because they are already tightly contracted. This condition is often best treated by pelvic floor physical therapy performed by a qualified pelvic floor physical therapist.

Basic pelvic muscle exercises are often called Kegel exercises, named for Arnold Kegel, the physician who first developed them. Regular Kegel exercises may be helpful particularly for women with mild to moderate stress incontinence. Learning to perform a strong and fast pelvic muscle contraction just before and during actions that commonly cause problems for those with stress incontinence (such as coughing or jumping) reduces leakage. Pelvic muscle exercises may also help overactive bladder and mixed incontinence.

For men, Kegels can help prevent post-void dribbling (see "Dribble relief," page 31). But studies have not shown Kegel exercises alone to be particularly effective in preventing or treating incontinence that results from prostate surgery.

Because Kegels cost nothing and are quite safe, they are recommended for most patients, either alone or in combination with other treatments. In essence, Kegels simply involve finding your pelvic floor muscles and then repeatedly contracting and relaxing them. Here's how to do Kegels correctly.

Locate your pelvic muscles. Pretend you are trying to avoid passing gas. If you are a woman, you can pretend to tighten your vagina around a tampon. Both actions involve the pelvic muscles. You will feel a correct contraction more in the back than the front, like you are pulling the anal area in or stopping gas from escaping. This approach makes it easier to use the correct muscles than older advice to attempt stopping (or pretend to stop) your urine stream.

Choose your position. You can start by lying on your back until you get the feel of contracting the pelvic floor muscles. Later, you can practice while sitting or standing as well.

Practice contractions. Practice both short contractions and releases (sometimes called "quick flicks") and longer ones (gradually increasing the strength of the contraction and holding it at your maximum for up to 10 seconds).

Relax between contractions. Consciously relax the muscles between each repetition, and hold the relaxation phase for the same amount of time as the contraction.

Keep other muscles relaxed. When doing pelvic floor exercises, don't push out your abdominal muscles, contract your leg or buttock muscles, or lift your pelvis. Rest a hand gently on your belly to detect unwanted abdominal action.

Repetitions. Your health professional may advise you how many Kegel exercises to do. It is more effective to spread the exercises throughout the day than to do them all at once. One simple starting regimen is to do 10 before getting out of bed, 10 standing after lunch, 10 in the evening while sitting watching TV, and another 10 before going to sleep. You can do them at other times as well: in the car sitting at a stoplight, waiting for an elevator, or waiting in a grocery line.

Determine your strategy. You can practice using these exercises to control your symptoms. If you have stress incontinence, tighten your pelvic floor muscles just before lifting, coughing, laughing, or whatever usually causes urine leakage. Do the same several times when you have the urge to urinate and doubt you are going to make it to the toilet. This should enable you to maintain control while you walk to the toilet.

Be consistent. Practice consistently, using whatever schedule works for you. It may take a few months for you to notice an improvement in your symptoms.

Pelvic floor physical therapy

Your physician may recommend that you see a physical therapist with training in pelvic floor therapy. Many people find it useful to have a trained expert help them identify the proper muscles and teach them to perform exercises correctly. A physical therapist trained in this specialty can also use biofeedback to aid in the process or electrical stimulation to help strengthen weak muscles.

Body posture, also known as body mechanics, is another important part of keeping pelvic floor muscles and structures functioning as they should. Maintaining the correct posture while you are doing exercises can ensure you are working the proper muscles, and in everyday life sitting or standing without slumping helps reduce pressure on the pelvic floor.

In addition, a physical therapist with specialty training can advise a patient on bladder training and lifestyle modifications and can provide regular rein-

▶ **Strike a pose**

Women with stress incontinence often dread forms of high-impact exercise that can result in leakage. In contrast, yoga exercises may actually improve incontinence. In a 2014 study of middle-aged and older women, those who took a six-week yoga class reduced their episodes of incontinence 70%, compared with a 13% reduction in women who received a booklet of self-help strategies but no yoga training. The yoga class used the Iyengar technique, a form that emphasizes safety and precise alignment and uses props to accommodate people who are less strong and flexible. During 90-minute classes twice a week, the women were taught eight yoga poses, with the instructors emphasizing how to become aware of and strengthen their pelvic floor muscles. In addition, they practiced at least one hour each week on their own. While the biggest improvement was in stress incontinence, the stress relief yoga can bring may ease overactive bladder symptoms as well. Note that this was a small study of only 19 women. Larger studies are needed to know for sure if yoga actually helps reduce incontinence.

forcement and advice. Not all physical therapists have expertise in bladder training, so ask about it before you begin your physical therapy sessions.

Using biofeedback to learn pelvic floor exercises

Both men and women can make use of biofeedback, a technique that uses a device to detect information about a biological function (for example, heart rate, skin temperature, or muscle tension) and provides feedback so you can gain greater awareness and control over that function. Biofeedback is performed by a trained practitioner such as a licensed physical therapist. Home biofeedback units are also available.

In the case of incontinence, biofeedback can help you identify pelvic floor muscles and learn to strengthen and control them in order to lessen stress incontinence, overactive bladder, and mixed incontinence.

For a biofeedback session, the practitioner inserts a small monitor into your vagina or rectum, or both. Electrodes may also be pasted on your belly to monitor abdominal contractions. As you perform your assigned pelvic exercises, you watch a computer screen and see a line or image (such as clouds or birds) rising as you contract the correct muscles more strongly. Some people have a single training session using biofeedback, while others go for six or more sessions spread over several weeks.

Devices are available to help you do pelvic muscle exercises consistently and effectively at home. Research shows home biofeedback devices yield comparable results to vaginal weighted cones (see page 19). But many pieces of equipment sold via the Internet for urinary incontinence have not been tested for effectiveness. For example, exercise contraptions that you squeeze between your legs generally do not work because they don't exercise the right muscles.

Home biofeedback devices. These handheld electronic devices let you know how strongly you are contracting your pelvic muscles when you practice Kegels. FDA-approved systems (such as Myself or the PFX Pelvic Floor Exerciser) are available without a prescription. Muscle strength is detected with a vaginal sensor and displayed on the handheld component; the PFX device is also available in a men's model that uses an anal probe. In other systems, you buy a vaginal probe and rent the biofeedback device by the month.

Vaginal weighted cones. Some women find that using vaginal weighted cones helps boost the power of their pelvic floor exercises. These are a set of smooth, tampon-shaped inserts of increasing weight. If you have significant uterine prolapse or a vaginal wall prolapse, your doctor will probably not recommend this method for strengthening your pelvic muscles.

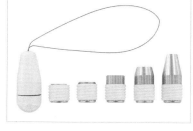

Vaginal weighted cones.

To use vaginal cones, start with the lightest (less than an ounce) and insert the cone into your vagina as you would a tampon. A lubricant may make insertion more comfortable, but it also makes the cone slippery. Then, contract your pelvic muscles to hold it in place. If contracting your muscles pushes the cone out, it may not be inserted far enough, or you may be pushing out with your abdominal muscles.

Vaginal cones function both as a strengthening tool and as a simple biofeedback device. If the cone stays in, you're contracting your muscles correctly. Start with three to five minutes, twice a day. Work up to 15 minutes, twice a day. Once you can hold a cone in place while walking, coughing, or going up and down stairs, switch to the next heavier cone.

A 2013 Cochrane review found evidence that the use of vaginal cones is helpful and may be similarly effective to electrical stimulation (see below) or pelvic floor muscle training, without requiring that you do specific exercises or be instructed in how to perform the contractions correctly.

Electrical stimulation

Some men and women find that they are unable to exercise their pelvic muscles consistently or effectively, or would appreciate help in beginning to condition the muscles. Often called "electro-stim," this method can be used to strengthen muscles to improve stress incontinence or to help relax the bladder muscle to improve overactive bladder.

Men and women can use either a portable device at home (such as the over-the-counter Apex or the prescription-only Pathway STM-10) or a larger system in a health professional's office. A small electrode, placed inside a woman's vagina or a man's or woman's rectum, delivers an electrical current that can spur your pelvic muscles to contract painlessly. You will feel as though you are doing a Kegel. The instruments can be set for different strengths of stimulation and various time intervals of contraction and relaxation. It is recommended that a nurse or health professional trained in pelvic floor disorders teach you how to use the device correctly.

For stress incontinence, electrical stimulation is believed to work by strengthening the muscle. For overactive bladder, a different frequency may help reset your nervous system's control over the bladder muscle. Medicare will cover some of the cost of renting a pelvic muscle stimulation device if it is prescribed by your physician and you can document that you have tried standard pelvic muscle exercises for four weeks and not gotten relief.

Medication to treat urinary incontinence

Certain drugs occasionally help with stress incontinence, though none are specifically approved for this purpose. Medications can be very helpful for overactive bladder and are also used for nocturia and overflow incontinence (see Table 2, page 20). In men who have overflow incontinence caused by an enlarged prostate, medications to shrink the prostate may help. Work with your health care provider to find the medication that results in the fewest side effects, at the lowest dose that eases symptoms. This may take some trial and error.

Before starting any new medication, inform your doctor about any other drugs you are taking. Some medications may be unsafe or ineffective when combined with an incontinence medication. Before prescribing a medication for incontinence, your doctor will also want to make certain that no other drug you are taking could be causing your incontinence (see Table 1, page 8). If so, changing that prescription

Table 2: Medications for urinary incontinence

GENERIC NAME	BRAND NAME(S)	USE IN INCONTINENCE	SIDE EFFECTS
Alpha-adrenergic antagonists			
alfuzosin	Uroxatral	For men with enlarged prostate: relax bladder neck muscles in men with obstructions.	Low blood pressure upon standing up, dizziness, lack of energy, swollen ankles.
doxazosin	Cardura		
tamsulosin	Flomax		
terazosin	Hytrin		
Antibiotics			
nitrofurantoin	Macrobid	For sudden-onset incontinence due to infection: may cure the problem.	Side effects vary by drug, but may include nausea, vomiting, sun sensitivity, rash, and jaundice. Do not take nitrofurantoin if you have liver or kidney problems.
sulfamethoxazole combined with trimethoprim	Bactrim, Septra		
many others	many others		
Anticholinergics			
darifenacin	Enablex	For overactive bladder: quiet bladder muscle spasms to ease urgency and frequency.	Dry mouth, dry eyes, headache, constipation, blurred vision. Slow-release versions cause fewer side effects.
fesoterodine	Toviaz		
flavoxate	Urispas		
oxybutynin	Ditropan XL, Gelnique gel, Oxytrol patch		
solifenacin	Vesicare		
tolterodine tartrate	Detrol LA		
trospium	Sanctura, Sanctura XR		
Antidepressants (tricyclic)			
amitriptyline	Elavil	For overactive bladder, stress incontinence, and sometimes nocturia. Low doses may help.	Drowsiness, blurry vision, constipation, dry mouth. Many reactions with other medications.
imipramine	Tofranil		
Antidiuretic hormone			
desmopressin	DDAVP, Noctiva	For nocturia: reduces urine production at night.	Dizziness, headache, weakness, low sodium in blood.
Beta-3 adrenergic agonist			
mirabegron	Myrbetriq	For overactive bladder: relaxes bladder muscles.	Increased blood pressure, difficult urination, headache.
Cholinergic			
bethanechol	Duvoid, Urecholine	For overflow incontinence: strengthens bladder muscle contraction.	Shortness of breath, blurry vision, drowsiness.
Injectable neurotoxin			
botulinum toxin	Botox	For overactive bladder and bladder dysfunction caused by nerve damage. Effects last three to 12 months.	Urinary retention, urinary tract infection.

might solve the problem without introducing a new medication.

In addition to medication, your doctor may suggest you use Kegel exercises to improve the strength and control of your pelvic floor muscles, along with bladder training and other behavioral strategies to suppress urgency. In a 237-woman trial comparing the medication tolterodine given alone or with training in behavioral techniques, women receiving the combination achieved better bladder control and were more satisfied with their treatment. However, most were not able to discontinue their medication.

Following are some types of drugs that sometimes help with symptoms.

Alpha-adrenergic antagonists. Alpha-adrenergic antagonists, also known as alpha blockers, relax the smooth muscle of the urethra. These drugs are prescribed to men who develop overflow incontinence when an enlarged prostate interferes with normal urine flow. They include alfuzosin (Uroxatral), doxazosin (Cardura), tamsulosin (Flomax), and terazosin (Hytrin). Women should not take alpha-adrenergic antagonists unless prescribed by their doctor. Although these drugs can help with overflow incontinence in men, they can make women leakier because they relax the smooth muscle of the urethra.

Note: These medications lower blood pressure and may make you prone to a sudden drop in blood pressure when you change position from lying down to sitting or standing (called postural hypotension). To minimize this symptom, your doctor may suggest taking the medication at bedtime. Some doctors are hesitant to prescribe these alpha blockers for men who are already on another blood pressure medication. Other side effects may include dizziness, lack of energy, or swelling of the ankles.

If you are planning cataract surgery, tell your ophthalmologist if you are taking an alpha-adrenergic antagonist. The drugs can affect how the pupils of your eyes act during the procedure, which may necessitate a change in surgical technique.

Anticholinergics. For women, anticholinergics are the mainstay of treatment for overactive bladder. These drugs block the effects of the neurotransmitter acetylcholine, which causes the detrusor muscle to contract. They are used to quiet the spasms of the bladder muscle that cause frequency, urgency, and urge incontinence.

Anticholinergics such as darifenacin (Enablex), fesoterodine (Toviaz), oxybutynin (Ditropan XL and others), solifenacin (Vesicare), tolterodine tartrate (Detrol LA), and trospium (Sanctura XR) are available in an extended-release form that minimizes side effects. Oxybutynin is also available in topical applications applied to the skin by patch or in gel form.

Note: Some people taking the drugs experience side effects such as dry mouth and dry eyes, headache, constipation, and blurred vision. Some older users report memory problems, and the drugs may worsen dementia. To avoid that, if you are older or have started to develop memory problems, your doctor may prescribe trospium, an anticholinergic that does not cross the blood-brain barrier. Talk to your doctor if you experience side effects or don't get the results you expect. You may need to try more than one medication to find the one that works best and causes the fewest side effects. About 80% of people are able to tolerate one of these drugs—a big improvement over older anticholinergics. You should not use anticholinergics if you have narrow-angle glaucoma, myasthenia gravis, or severe ulcerative colitis. Men should not use the drugs to relieve symptoms in lieu of getting a proper prostate evaluation.

Antidepressants. An older category of antidepressant drugs known as tricyclic antidepressants, such as amitriptyline (Elavil) and imipramine (Tofranil), can be useful for treating men and women whose primary complaint is that they wake up frequently at night to urinate (a condition called nocturia). Because these antidepressants cause drowsiness and relax the bladder muscle, they can help people sleep through the night. Low doses are sometimes prescribed either alone or in combination with anticholinergics to treat overactive bladder.

Note: Tricyclic antidepressants interact with a number of common medications, so your physician should be aware of all the medications you use (including over-the-counter or alternative remedies) before prescribing them. Antidepressants such as fluoxetine (Prozac), in the class known as selective serotonin reuptake inhibitors (SSRIs), are not effective in treating incontinence.

Antidiuretic hormone. This synthetic hormone can be useful for men or women who are primarily troubled by the need to urinate during the night because of increased urine production at night. Normally vasopressin, an antidiuretic hormone produced by the pituitary gland, signals the kidneys to reduce urine production while you sleep. The synthetic version, desmopressin (DDAVP, Noctiva), works the same way.

Note: If you have a medical condition that would be worsened by fluid retention (such as high blood pressure or heart failure), your doctor is unlikely to prescribe antidiuretic hormone. Your electrolytes need to be carefully monitored when starting this medication, as it can cause dangerously low levels of sodium in your blood.

Beta-3 adrenergic agonist. Extended-release mirabegron (Myrbetriq)—the first drug of its kind—relaxes bladder muscles to prevent urinary urgency, frequency, and incontinence. It is taken daily, with food or without. Mirabegron provides an alternative treatment for overactive bladder for those who can't tolerate the side effects of anticholinergic medications, such as dry eye and dry mouth, or if anticholinergic medication does not help.

Note: Uncommon side effects of this drug can include an increase in blood pressure, difficult urination, and headache. Your insurer may not cover mirabegron unless you have previously tried two or more anticholinergics.

Cholinergic. The cholinergic drug bethanechol (sold as Duvoid, Urecholine, or in generic form) strengthens the contractions of the bladder muscle and may be prescribed to men and women who have overflow incontinence because of a weak bladder muscle (not a blockage). Side effects can include shortness of breath, blurry vision, sweating, and dizziness. The medication is usually taken an hour or two before meals to prevent stomach upset.

Note: You should not take bethanechol if you have asthma, an overactive thyroid, or Parkinson's disease, or if you have recently had surgery on your urinary system or gastrointestinal tract.

Estrogen. Estrogen is sometimes prescribed as a vaginal supplement to improve the strength of tissues in the urinary tract of women who show signs of deficiency. It may also help relieve symptoms of urinary frequency and urgency incontinence. However, in the large multicenter trial known as the Women's Health Initiative, oral conjugated equine estrogen (Premarin), both alone and combined with a progestin (in a drug called Prempro, the most commonly prescribed formulation), worsened stress incontinence and overactive bladder in postmenopausal women who already had incontinence, and increased the risk that incontinence would develop in women who were continent at the beginning of the study. A 2012 Cochrane review found some evidence that vaginal estrogen therapy can reduce urgency and episodes of urinary incontinence.

Note: Hormone therapy is generally recommended only for the short-term treatment of menopausal symptoms. However, using vaginal estrogen in the form of a cream, a ring, or suppositories one to three times a week is safe over the long term because the estrogen does not enter the bloodstream in significant amounts.

Stimulation devices for overactive bladder

Without your awareness, there is a constant loop of communication between your bladder and one of your lower spinal nerves (the third sacral nerve). About six times per second, the sacral nerve sends an impulse to the bladder to remind it "don't go now." If that signal isn't sufficiently strong or frequent, you can develop problems with urgency and frequency, known as overactive bladder. Certain devices and strategies aim to improve the signaling from this sacral nerve by using low-level electrical stimulation.

Sacral nerve stimulation

In the late 1990s, the FDA approved a pacemaker-like implanted device for use in men and women with bladder overactivity that has not responded to medication, bladder training, or biofeedback. Since that time, the use of this device has grown more common. If your doctor thinks the device might help you, you can be temporarily fitted with a test system. To do so, the physician places a wire near your sacral nerve and attaches it to an external device that sends electrical impulses through it. This is done either in the physician's office or in the operating room under light, intravenous sedation. If your symptoms improve by more than 50% while wearing the device, you are a good candidate for long-term stimulation.

The long-term device is inserted surgically while you are under general or local anesthesia. The surgeon makes a small incision over the sacrum (the spinal bone above your tailbone) and inserts a lead wire there. From the sacrum, the wire runs just under your skin and fat layer until it connects to the small stimulator device (about the size of a stopwatch) implanted just under the skin and fat in an unobtrusive location in your upper buttock or abdomen. You use a handheld control device to adjust the stimulator as necessary. About every five years, you will need another minor surgery to replace the battery.

Note: This treatment is not without risks. Within the first six months, about 4% of patients require repeat surgery because of pain, infection, or movement of the wire. The manufacturer warns that while the device is in place, it is unsafe to undergo medical treatments involving diathermy (heating parts of the body using electrical currents or ultrasound); the energy can damage the system and cause serious or life-threatening damage to surrounding tissue. In addition, with limited exceptions for head examinations, MRI is not recommended for people with a sacral nerve stimulation device.

This treatment is expensive, but Medicare and most insurers cover it.

Percutaneous tibial nerve stimulation

Another way to access the nerves that help control your bladder is through a nerve located in your ankle. (The ankle and the bladder receive signals from the same sacral nerve.) For a percutaneous tibial nerve stimulation (PTNS) treatment, which lasts about half an hour, a hair-thin wire is inserted near the tibial nerve just above your ankle. The wire is connected to an external device that delivers low-frequency electrical pulses. The stimulation travels to the sacral nerve, where it is designed to reset nerve signals to the bladder and thus diminish incontinence related to an overactive bladder. The treatment is used once a week for 12 weeks and then as needed (often once or twice a month) for maintenance to control symptoms. In one U.S. multicenter study, 12 weeks of PTNS treatment cured or improved 80% of patients, compared with 61% of a control group who were prescribed medication (tolterodine).

Note: You may not be able to use this treatment if you are pregnant or have certain conditions (such as nerve damage). PTNS for urinary incontinence is often covered by Medicare and other insurers.

Injections

Rather than taking medications, which affect the whole body, some people gain relief through local injections that prevent unwanted muscle contractions or provide added support to pelvic structures.

Botulinum toxin

Best known for its ability to smooth a furrowed brow by paralyzing forehead muscles, botulinum toxin A (Botox) is sometimes used to relieve severe overactive bladder in people either unable to tolerate or not responding to lifestyle modifications, bladder training, pelvic floor physical therapy, or medication. Either in the office or at an outpatient surgery center, your physician passes a cystoscope through the urethra into the bladder, then injects the toxin directly into the detrusor muscle in many locations, where it weakens the muscle's ability to contract.

Note: Botulinum toxin runs the risk of causing the opposite problem from the one you are trying to treat—it can lead to temporary urinary retention, or the inability to urinate. To avoid this, it is recommended that a physician begin by injecting a low starting dose and switching to a higher dose if needed to obtain the desired effect. Injections of botulinum toxin usually need to be repeated every three to 12 months, as the effects wear off.

Bulking agents for stress incontinence

Injection of a bulking agent can reinforce the tissue around the urethra. This procedure can help some men who have had their prostate removed and some women with the type of stress incontinence known as urethral incompetence, in which the urinary sphincter no longer closes completely and allows urine to leak out, particularly with exertion. The bulking agent keeps the urethra tighter so that it stays closed against increased pressure.

Available injectables include calcium hydroxylapatite particles suspended in gel (Coaptite) and a silicone-containing product (Macroplastique). The life span of synthetic bulking agents is unknown, but they have been demonstrated to remain for at least a year.

Injection of bulking agents takes 10 to 30 minutes and can be performed in the physician's office or as an outpatient procedure in the hospital. Using a cystoscope for viewing, the doctor places a needle into the urethra and injects the bulking agent into the tissue alongside the urethra. A few injections may be given during one session. You will usually be given just local anesthesia. Only small amounts of bulking agents are injected at one time, so more than one treatment may be needed to achieve satisfactory results. Physicians must be cautious about injecting too much, as this can cause inability to urinate.

For the first day or two after an injection, you may feel irritation when you urinate. You might even need to use a catheter to drain the bladder intermittently until swelling goes down in the area of the injection. After a few days, you should be able to return to normal activities.

Bulking agents work best in women with urethral incompetence; they are not likely to help if you have overactive bladder, an abnormally small bladder capacity, or a bladder neck that is not well supported. In general, bulking agents are most useful for older women who do not do strenuous physical activity and who may not be good candidates for other treatments. They don't work as well as other methods, particularly in people who are physically active. About 80% of women show some level of improvement; 40% become dry and remain dry with only one or two treatments. Women should not be injected with bulking agents if they currently have a urinary tract infection or if the physician sees through the cystoscope that the lining of the urethra is fragile and might erode in the area of the injection.

Some men have this procedure after prostate removal; the bulking agent is injected into the area the prostate had occupied in order to provide support for the urethral muscles, so urine isn't as easily lost. Although 70% of men experience some improvement in their symptoms, only 8% become dry with one or two treatments and require no further injections.

Surgery

The trend in surgery for incontinence is toward less invasive surgical procedures that can usually be performed on an outpatient basis and sometimes in the physician's office. Because some surgical procedures for stress incontinence are now relatively quick and require less recovery time, your doctor may recommend surgery earlier if your incontinence is caused by a repairable structural problem or if it seems unlikely that nonsurgical approaches will be satisfactory. When choosing to have minimally invasive surgery, it is especially important that your surgeon be highly trained and experienced in the specific procedure you choose (see "Selecting your procedure and surgeon," page 25).

The most common condition treated surgically is stress incontinence; this is done by inserting a sling of material to support the urethra. Overactive bladder may also be treated with the surgical implantation of a device that regularly stimulates the sacral nerve (see "Sacral nerve stimulation," page 22). If incontinence is caused by an enlarged prostate in a man, surgery to correct that condition may relieve the incontinence along with other symptoms.

Whether and when to have surgery is a personal decision that has no right or wrong answer. You might consider surgery if nonsurgical treatments are not providing the control you need or if an anatomical problem makes it unlikely that nonsurgical techniques will help. Even if surgery is ultimately your choice, the effort you spend in bladder training and strengthening your pelvic muscles is not wasted; these techniques increase the chance of a successful outcome following surgery for incontinence and can reduce postoperative incontinence after prostate surgery. After their operations, some people say they regret the time they spent coping with incontinence and wish they had taken the step sooner. Others hope to put off the decision as long as possible, because new and less invasive procedures are becoming available every year.

Surgery for stress incontinence

For women, surgeries for stress incontinence are designed to provide extra support for the urethra so it can remain closed under physical stress, such as during coughing or sneezing. This can be done by several methods. For years, the best method was the Burch procedure, a form of bladder neck suspension in which the surgeon places stitches on either side of the urethra and bladder neck and attaches the stitches to a ligament at the top of the pubic bone. Another procedure involves a simple-to-install sling of synthetic mesh that supports the urethra, hammock-style.

Before you and your doctor decide on surgery, you may need to have detailed diagnostic testing to help determine which type of surgery would work best. The availability of minimally invasive procedures has led physicians to consider such treatments for stress incontinence in women who are younger and have less severe incontinence as well as older women who may benefit from a minimally invasive procedure. However, women who hope to have future pregnancies are often advised to postpone surgery if possible until childbearing is complete, because delivering a baby through the vaginal canal may undo the effects of the surgery. If you do opt for surgery, choose your surgeon and procedure carefully, because additional attempts may be less successful (see "Selecting your procedure and surgeon," at left).

Before your surgery, gain the best control possible over your bladder by strengthening your pelvic floor, using bladder training, and avoiding bladder irritants such as caffeine. This will minimize urinary urgency and frequency, which can develop following surgery.

Three distressing but uncommon problems may occur after any type of surgery for stress incontinence, although the risks vary with the different procedures:

- You might develop symptoms of overactive bladder, even if you were never troubled by them before (7% to 15% of patients experience this).
- Although it's not common, you might undo the benefits of the surgery by lifting or other strenuous activity, even after the healing period is over.
- You might go from incontinence to having difficulty urinating, in some cases requiring a catheter temporarily to empty your bladder.

Sling procedures. These procedures have become increasingly common because they are less invasive and just as effective as older surgical methods, such as the Burch procedure. For these operations, a surgeon installs a mesh sling under and around the urethra to support it. The sling is made of either your own tissue or of polypropylene, a material similar to nylon that has been used as suture material for many years. In

---

Selecting your procedure and surgeon

If you are planning surgery for urinary incontinence, you may have several choices of procedures. Among the factors in your decision will be the risks and benefits of each option and the specific problems your evaluation has revealed. In addition, you and your physician may favor one approach over another for individual reasons. Among things to consider:

- Is a rapid recovery and return to work a priority?

- Do you need another pelvic surgery—such as a hysterectomy, tubal ligation, or treatment for prolapse—that can be done at the same time? (This could be done by either two surgeons in coordination or a urogynecologist who can perform both procedures.)

- Are you more comfortable using your own tissue or a synthetic material?

Remember, not all surgeons may be prepared to offer the least invasive option suitable to your medical situation. Look for a urologist or urogynecologist who has substantial experience in urinary procedures and is up to date with the latest approaches. A good place to start may be the provider locator on the website of the American Urogynecologic Society or its patient website, Voices for PFD (see "Resources," page 47): both urologists and urogynecologists belong to the group. Before agreeing to the surgery, ask the surgeon how often he or she performs the particular procedure. If you have any concerns about the surgeon's experience, or still have questions about whether a particular procedure is right for you, seek a second opinion.

---

women, the sling provides a backstop for the urethra to press against during a cough or sneeze, helping to hold in urine. In men, the sling puts pressure on the urethra just below the bladder.

After minimally invasive surgery such as this, recovery is rapid. If you are over age 70 or have other medical problems, you may be hospitalized overnight. Otherwise, you will probably be discharged after you have recovered from any anesthesia and have been able to urinate. If you are not able to urinate adequately, you may go home with a Foley catheter (small tube) to drain your bladder for one to three days. If you go home with a catheter, usually you will return to the doctor's office to have the catheter removed by a nurse. You may need pain relief medication for a few days. Initially your urine stream may be slower. When you sit to urinate, relax and wait for the reflex that starts urine flowing. Straining can make it more difficult to urinate and can loosen the sling.

Note: In 2011, the FDA issued a safety recommendation warning doctors and their female patients about the use of mesh to treat pelvic organ prolapse. However, the use of the mesh in pelvic organ prolapse is very different from the use of sling procedures for urinary incontinence. In pelvic organ prolapse, larger pieces of mesh are inserted through the vaginal canal and affixed to tissue next to the vaginal canal. These mesh pieces sometimes shrink and pull on tissues, resulting in complications such as erosion of the vaginal wall, pain, and bleeding. The FDA, after looking at the data, has not issued a warning about mesh when used for urinary incontinence. If you are considering any sling procedures, the key to a successful, complication-free outcome is choosing an experienced surgeon who performs the procedure frequently.

Slings for women. Several types of minimally invasive sling surgery are available. Depending on your symptoms, your surgeon may recommend one type of sling over another.

- In a mid-urethral sling procedure, the surgeon places a hammock of narrow mesh underneath the urethra and extending up the abdominal wall behind the pubic bone, forming a U-shape to support the urethra (see Figure 6, at left; the U-shape isn't obvious in the side view, but is clear when seen from the front). The mesh stays in place without sutures, as your body's tissues grow through the mesh. This surgery is faster and easier than older, more invasive sling procedures and, in many cases, can be performed under local anesthesia. Some surgeons combine the placement of a mid-urethral sling with other pelvic reconstructive surgery, such as vaginal hysterectomy or repair of anterior or posterior vaginal prolapse (cystocele or rectocele). Most women can return to work within three to seven days after a mid-urethral sling procedure as long as their jobs do not require heavy lifting.

- In an obturator sling procedure, the sling is inserted through a small vaginal incision, and the ends are brought out through tiny incisions between the labia and the crease of the thighs, so the sling forms a curve shaped more like a smile than the letter U. No sutures are necessary. Surgery takes about half an hour, and most women can return to work within a few days if they do not have to lift heavy objects. Because it does not involve abdominal incisions, the obturator sling procedure reduces the risk of bowel or bladder injury during surgery.

Figure 6: Sling surgery (for women)

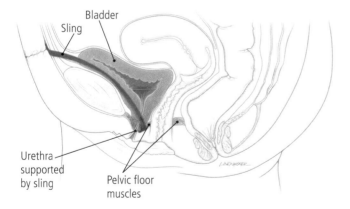

For some women with stress incontinence (leaking when coughing or jumping), the surgical insertion of a urethral sling can help support the urethra. In the version shown here, known as a mid-urethral sling procedure, the surgeon makes a small incision under the urethra through the vagina and two small incisions in the lower abdomen, to insert a strip of synthetic mesh under the urethra to support it. Gradually, your body's own tissues grow through the mesh to hold it in place.

- In a single-incision sling procedure, called the mini sling, the surgeon inserts a supportive mesh hammock under the urethra using a slim needle. The procedure requires a small vaginal incision but no abdominal or groin incisions, and it may be performed in an outpatient surgery center or a physician's office under local anesthesia. Since the mini sling was introduced in 2007, several studies have examined its effectiveness. When combined results were analyzed from nine trials involving 758 women, during an average of 9.5 months of follow-up, the mini slings provided less improvement and required more reoperations than standard sling procedures. More recently, in a study with a follow-up period of 20 to 29 months, 86% of 51 women who received the Ajust mini sling experienced improved or restored continence.

In all sling procedures, it is important that patients follow postoperative instructions to avoid excessive activity, such as lifting or exercise, during the healing process. After the surgery, there is a possibility that the sling will push too hard against the urethra, blocking the flow of urine. If this occurs, a second, minor surgery may be necessary to loosen up the sling. Some people develop symptoms of urinary urgency (even if this was never a problem previously) that can usually be controlled with medication, bladder training, or Kegel exercises. Rarely, the mesh sling may erode into the vaginal canal or other tissues. These problems can usually be corrected with either vaginal estrogen or further surgery.

Slings for men. Minimally invasive sling surgery (also called bulbourethral sling surgery) is relatively simple and usually does not require an overnight hospital stay. During the half-hour procedure, which is performed under spinal or general anesthesia, the surgeon makes an incision between the scrotum and rectum and attaches the sling to anchors or screws inserted into each side of the pelvic bone.

Complications following male sling procedures can include infection, discomfort, and a shift from incontinence to the opposite problems—urinary retention or difficulty urinating. Men may need to use a catheter to empty their bladders for a short time after this surgery. The sling is usually for men who have mild to moderate stress incontinence due to prostate removal or treatment, other surgery, or trauma. Scarring from previous surgeries or injuries (such as a pelvic fracture) may decrease the likelihood of success.

Bladder neck suspension. Known as the Burch colposuspension, bladder neck suspension is a surgical procedure for women with stress incontinence that elevates or increases support for the bladder neck area to protect against leakage when a woman coughs or exerts herself physically. This operation often involves cutting an incision of three to five inches in the lower abdomen and lifting the tissue next to the bladder neck up, using strong stitches (sutures) to anchor the tissue to a ligament (called Cooper's ligament) near the pubic bone. The Burch procedure is performed under general anesthesia and usually requires a two-day hospital stay and six weeks of recovery before a woman can return to full activity. Sometimes the procedure can be performed laparoscopically, with a quicker recovery.

Figure 7: Artificial urinary sphincter (for men)

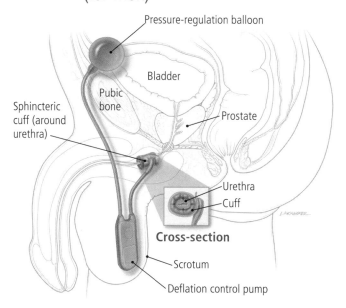

For men who have had prostate surgery, initial incontinence usually improves over several months. But for those with intractable incontinence caused by sphincter weakness, the artificial sphincter is a possible solution. After it is surgically inserted, the fluid-filled cuff compresses the urethra to stop the flow of urine. To allow urination, a man squeezes a small pump to open the cuff and allow urine to pass. The cuff automatically refills.

Surgery for severe stress incontinence

If your problem is severe, simple sling procedures or bladder neck suspension will not be sufficient. However, you have other options.

Artificial urinary sphincter. An artificial sphincter is a fluid-filled cuff surgically placed around the urethra to prevent urine from leaking out (see Figure 7, page 27). A small pump is inserted into the scrotum in a man or one of the labia (the tissue surrounding and protecting the openings of the vagina and urethra) in a woman. To urinate, you squeeze the pump and the fluid drains from the cuff into a storage balloon implanted in the abdominal cavity. This releases pressure on the urethra and allows urine to flow out. Over the next few minutes, the fluid automatically returns to the cuff.

The operation to implant the cuff, balloon, and pump takes about two hours and three small incisions. It is usually performed under general anesthesia. During a healing period of four to six weeks, the pump will not be activated. Once the pump is activated, your urinary control will improve. The major complications with an artificial sphincter include the possibility of infection, erosion of the tissue around the implants, or malfunctioning or shifting of the device. Such complications may require surgery to repair or remove the device.

Artificial sphincters are used far less frequently in women than in men. However, if you are a woman with severe stress incontinence due to urethral incompetence, or if you are still having major leakage problems after other surgeries, the artificial sphincter is an option.

Suprapubic tube insertion. For severe and intractable incontinence, a surgeon can insert a suprapubic (above the pubic bone) tube from outside your abdomen directly into your bladder. Urine is diverted through the tube and collected in a bag outside the body. Although this solution is a last resort, it is easier than other management techniques for people in some situations. Although for the average person this would mean a reduced quality of life, for those with truly severe incontinence, it can be a big improvement.

Surgery for overflow incontinence

If you have overflow incontinence because something is blocking your urethra (such as an enlarged prostate in a man), surgery can be performed to remove the obstruction. The procedures and results will depend on the exact cause and location of the blockage.

For example, a man with an enlarged prostate may undergo transurethral resection of the prostate, or TURP, an incision-free surgical procedure that removes excess prostate tissue through the penis. It relieves urinary obstruction in at least 75% of cases, and the improvement is usually long-lasting. However, urinary problems can recur if the prostate tissue grows back. While TURP may aid overflow incontinence, other types of incontinence may occur as a side effect of the procedure. (For more detailed information on surgeries for benign prostatic hyperplasia, see the *Annual Report on Prostate Diseases* from Harvard Medical School. Ordering information is in the "Resources" section, page 47.)

Women with incontinence resulting from a prolapsed bladder, uterus, or rectum may undergo procedures to reposition the out-of-place organs and shore up their support. ◗

Coping with urinary incontinence

Many people must cope with urinary incontinence— at least for a while before treatment, and sometimes afterward as well, if treatment does not completely correct the symptoms. If you are experiencing urinary incontinence, even temporarily, it's important to realize that you have other options beyond the expensive pads and "adult diapers" available on drugstore shelves. There are options designed specifically for men or women as well as pad-and-pants systems tailored to specific types of incontinence.

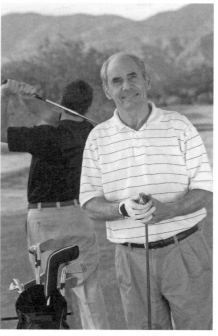

Don't let fear of leaks keep you from staying active. There are many ways to cope with urinary incontinence.

If you must deal with incontinence, seek advice from health professionals or support organizations such as the National Association for Continence (see "Resources," page 47). You will find less expensive, more effective products and learn strategies to maximize your ability to work, travel, and participate in your favorite activities. You can also learn about ways to help prevent your problem from worsening (see "Lifestyle choices that may improve your symptoms," page 30).

Containment options

A tremendous variety of pads and other absorbent products are available to suit your sex and the severity of your incontinence. In general, products designated for "light" protection will absorb up to one cup; "moderate," up to two cups; and "heavy," up to three cups.

When choosing a pad, look for products specifically for incontinence that incorporate super-absorbent layers; these pull fluid away from the skin into the core of the pad, where it forms a gel that can't leak out. Look for such brand names as Depend, Poise, Tena, and Serenity. Check with your insurer about coverage for products to manage incontinence. If your insurance does not cover these products, some people find they can use less-expensive children's diapers.

For women. Products include a range of disposable and reusable pads and underwear. Among these are traditional and even fashionable underwear designs (brand names include Icon, DRC, and Wearever) with a special crotch that wicks urine away from the surface and stores it. If you are limited in movement and dexterity, ask about products that are designed for easy use by people with disabilities. Women with mild incontinence may use less expensive and readily available menstrual pads, reserving specific (more expen-

© Mike Watson Images | Thinkstock

Lifestyle choices that may improve your symptoms

Not all incontinence is avoidable. But there are some lifestyle changes that both reduce the risk of developing either urinary or fecal incontinence and may improve your symptoms if you already have such a condition.

Maintain a healthy weight. Particularly for women, obesity is linked with incontinence. In people who are overweight or obese, the pelvic floor muscles must support excess abdominal fat as well as the pelvic organs, which can lead to stress incontinence. In addition, obesity may place pressure on the bladder and interfere with its blood and nerve supply. Fat tissue itself may contribute to overactive bladder by altering the balance of chemical messengers between nerve cells. Weight loss, whether achieved through diet and exercise or through bariatric surgery, can sometimes improve incontinence without other treatment.

A connection between obesity and urinary incontinence is not as well documented in men. However, in one study of men with type 2 diabetes, those who participated in extensive lifestyle therapy lost 9.4% of their body weight and were 38% less likely to have incontinence one year later (compared with those who received support and education not focused on weight loss). In some surveys, obese men report more urinary tract symptoms, including urgency and nocturia, and they are more likely to require surgery for an enlarged prostate (a procedure that sometimes leads to incontinence).

For men as well as women, many surgeries to counter incontinence are less successful in those who are obese.

Don't smoke. Smoking nearly doubles the likelihood that a woman will develop stress incontinence, perhaps because it can lead to frequent and violent coughing. Compared with other incontinent women, female smokers develop incontinence at a younger age, despite having relatively stronger sphincter muscles. Nicotine has also been linked to urge incontinence. In studies involving men, current or former smoking is associated with several bothersome urinary symptoms, including urge incontinence, but the increase in risk (about 39%) is not as striking as that for stress incontinence in women.

Stay active. High-impact exercises (such as jumping jacks) or specific maneuvers (such as a golf swing) can elicit leakage if you have stress incontinence. But don't let fear of leaks keep you from being physically active. In the Nurses' Health Study, middle-aged women who were most physically active were least likely to develop incontinence.

Cut back on caffeine and alcohol. Caffeine is a diuretic that results in rapid filling of the bladder and a powerful urge to urinate, even when the bladder is not full. Drinking just two cups of coffee per day has been linked to a higher risk of urinary incontinence. Like caffeine, alcohol is a diuretic that can create the urge to urinate.

Minimize bladder irritants. Several foods have been linked to urge incontinence. Carbonated drinks, the artificial sweetener aspartame (NutraSweet), spicy foods, and citrus fruits and juices cause urgency in some people.

Don't ignore the call. When you get your body's signal that the rectum is full, it's normal to wait until you can conveniently reach a bathroom. But when you routinely put off having a bowel movement as long as possible, it can lead to constipation and ultimately to urinary or fecal incontinence.

Don't strain with bowel movements. Years of forcing can weaken a man's or a woman's pelvic floor muscles. Even when you have regular bowel movements, if your stools are frequently hard or take considerable effort to pass, you have constipation and could benefit from medical advice. Increasing the fiber in your diet and drinking adequate fluids can help prevent constipation. In a study involving people ages 65 and older, treating constipation improved a variety of urinary symptoms, including frequency, urgency, and burning.

Consider the risk of incontinence when making medical decisions. When you are considering any type of pelvic or abdominal surgery, such as a hysterectomy, prostate removal, or treatment for hemorrhoids (painful swellings in the anus) or anal fistula (a painful crack or slit in the anus), ask about the risk for subsequent incontinence from the proposed procedure and its alternatives. For example, prostate removal may result in urinary stress incontinence (an estimated 14% of men still have frequent urine leakage five years after the procedure), but alternative treatment with radiation seed therapy may cause urge incontinence, and external beam radiation can lead to bowel problems, including fecal incontinence. When a medication is prescribed, inquire about incontinence as a possible side effect and whether alternatives are available if symptoms occur.

If you are pregnant, ask your obstetrician about how often episiotomies are used in vaginal deliveries in that practice, and under what circumstances. If episiotomy is used frequently or routinely, discuss your concerns about sphincter damage and seek another practitioner if needed.

Get help early. Early symptoms are a warning sign. Don't wait for symptoms to worsen. Report symptoms to your doctor. Ask to see a pelvic floor physical therapist who can work with you to strengthen or stabilize your pelvic floor muscles to regain bladder and bowel control and improve your quality of life.

sive) products for when they need extra protection and dryness. Before investing in a large quantity of incontinence pads, try smaller packages of several brands to see which works best for you.

For men. There are several absorbent products designed with the male anatomy in mind. Drip shields (with light protection) or guards (which absorb more) have waterproof backings. They slip over the head of the penis and can be kept in place with any relatively tight-fitting briefs. Some cover the scrotum as well and fit better if the penis is small or retracted. Brand names include Attends and Conveen. These products absorb 3 to 4 ounces of urine. When men with light incontinence compared four types of products, drip guards were the favored design for day and night use. For heavier incontinence, you can wear absorbent inserts, shaped to fit men (such as Depend and Dignity), inside your own underwear or special mesh briefs.

Collection devices

When there is constant leakage, devices that collect rather than absorb the urine can help to protect the skin. The National Association for Continence advises individuals to seek professional guidance in selecting the type and size that would work best for them. Otherwise, a person may conclude that a device is unsatisfactory when the problem may, in fact, lie in its fit or style.

For men. Men can choose from a variety of external devices. A condom catheter, also known as a "Texas catheter," is a soft sheath made of silicone or latex that fits over the penis like a regular condom, except that it attaches to a drain tube leading to a urine collection bag, usually worn on the leg. Some condom catheters are self-adhesive; others must be strapped on, held in place with a jockstrap, or taped on with adhesive strips. Some are reusable, and others, disposable.

The major concern in using a condom catheter is protecting your skin. Usually, you should clean and dry your penis and apply a moisture-protective cream before attaching a new condom catheter. Some men develop a sensitivity to latex and should choose a silicone version.

For women. A few urine collection pouches (such as the Hollister female urinary pouch external collection device) are designed to be held around the opening to the urethra with adhesive or suction. The end of the pouch is connected to a larger drainage bag so you can move around freely.

Dribble relief

Many men, young and old, are troubled by the dribbling of urine after the main stream has stopped and the bladder feels empty. Even if they wait a moment and shake the penis before zipping up, there can be embarrassing wet or stained trousers. At highest risk: men with enlarged prostates.

The medical term for this is post-micturition dribbling. It occurs when the muscles surrounding the urethra don't squeeze hard enough for it to empty completely, leaving a small pool of urine at a dip in the urethra behind the base of the penis. Within a few minutes, the urine dribbles out.

Try these approaches to avoid wet and stained trousers:

- Practice pelvic floor exercises to increase muscle strength.
- "Milk out" the last few drops of urine. Using the fingertips of one hand, start about an inch behind your scrotum, and gently press upward. Keep applying this pressure as you move your fingers toward the base of the penis under the scrotum. Repeat. This maneuver should move the pooled urine into the penis, where you can shake out the last few drops. With practice, you should be able to do this quickly and unobtrusively.

In women, dribbling can occur when a little urine gets trapped in the vagina, dripping out when you stand up from the toilet. Wipe inside the vagina before standing to see if this eliminates the dripping.

Clamps for men

For men, an alternative to pads or collection devices is a clamp placed around the base of the penis and tightened just enough to prevent urine from leaking. The device is designed as an inflatable ring or a foam-lined metal or plastic frame. Every couple of hours, you loosen the clamp to urinate and keep pressure from building up. Whether a clamp works will depend on whether you can adjust it to prevent leakage and still remain comfortable.

Note: If you have damaged skin on the penis, are physically unable to loosen the clamp yourself, or have nerve damage that might make it difficult for you to judge the clamp's tightness, you could damage the tissues of the penis and are better off choosing a different method. Penile clamps are available without a prescription (brand names include the Cunningham Clamp, Gyrx Squeezer, and Jackson Medical J Clamp), but may be covered by Medicare or your private insurer if ordered through your physician.

Clean intermittent catheterization

If you are a man or woman with overflow incontinence because your bladder muscles are weak or your bladder does not completely empty for other reasons, such as complications of surgery for incontinence, you may be able to manage the situation with intermittent self-catheterization. For this approach, you urinate normally every few hours, trying to empty your bladder as completely as possible. Next you insert a small tube (the catheter) through the urethra into the bladder to drain any remaining urine into the toilet.

Although it may sound difficult, this technique is a major advance for people who need temporary or permanent help urinating. The procedure is not usu-

ally painful, and you do not need to keep the catheter sterile or use gloves. Urinary tract infections can be a problem, but this technique poses a smaller risk than a permanent catheter would. Prelubricated, compact, and disposable catheters (SpeediCath Compact for women and SpeediCath Hydrophilic for men) are easy to carry and use with discretion in any toilet stall.

Pessaries and bladder support devices for women

For centuries, women have used a device called a pessary, placed inside the vagina to prevent urine leakage by supporting the urethra. Although it sounds old-fashioned and doesn't actually repair the problem, a pessary can mimic the benefit of a surgical bladder neck suspension and is a very practical solution for some women with prolapse that results in stress incontinence.

Pessaries are usually ring- or dish-shaped and are available only through a physician or other health care provider. The pessary, inserted in a manner similar to a contraceptive diaphragm, must be fitted by your health care provider to support the bladder neck properly when it is inserted. Your clinician may suggest you use a pessary while you wait for surgery. This device might also be an option if surgery is considered medically unsafe or unlikely to relieve your symptoms, if you develop stress incontinence while pregnant, or if you prefer a nonsurgical option.

But it's usually not helpful if you have overactive bladder. If you have a vaginal infection, that will have to be treated before you use a pessary.

Whether you find a pessary beneficial will depend largely on your anatomy. If your pessary fits properly (and it typically takes two or more tries to select the ideal size and style), it should not fall out during normal activities and should not interfere with regular urination or having a bowel movement. Some pessaries can be left in place during intercourse, although you may be more comfortable removing the device. A health professional can work with you until you are comfortable inserting it and removing it for cleaning. Some pessaries must be removed every few days; others can be left in place for several months and are removed for cleaning at regular medical visits.

As an alternative to a doctor-fitted pessary, a non-absorbent disposable urethral support called Poise Impressa was cleared by the FDA and became available in 2015. This over-the-counter device is inserted into the vagina like a tampon and presses against the urethra to keep it closed (think of stepping on a garden hose). The device is available in three sizes. Purchase a fitting kit first and start with the smallest size. If it falls out, go to the next size up. Don't push the Impressa too far into the vagina—it will be effective only if it is under the urethra. If you find that it isn't working, try pulling it out a little or pushing it in a little, using the directions and pictures in the instructions to guide you. Often it takes three to four weeks to figure out the correct size and placement. Inserted with an applicator and removed via a string, just like many tampons, these supports are intended for temporary use and should not be left in place for more than eight hours in a day.

If you have urine leakage only during a specific activity, such as jogging or tennis, you might get temporary urethral support by inserting a short, wide tampon, such as an O.B. Super Plus, into your vagina so that it is under the urethra (not too far back).

Skin care

When incontinence is ongoing, it can be a challenge to keep the skin clean and healthy. Skin irritation can be an annoyance in some people, but it may become a serious medical problem in others, who develop pressure sores. Urine is particularly irritating because it is acidic; this increases the possibility that you will develop open sores on your skin. You can avoid skin irritation with measures to properly cleanse, repair, and protect the skin.

In general, after each episode of incontinence, cleanse the area with tepid water or a gentle, nonalkaline soap or cleanser. Then protect the skin with a lotion or cream used to protect baby skin (such as Balmex)

Is your home making things worse?

Falling on the way to the bathroom can cause a fracture or other injury, particularly for someone with overactive bladder or someone who gets up at night to urinate.

One solution is a bedside commode. Other measures include installing grab bars and nonslip surfaces in the bathroom, wearing slippers or flat-soled shoes that grip well, and clearing throw rugs and obstacles from the path between your bed and the bathroom.

---

or specifically developed for incontinence (such as ComfortShield or Convatec). A Cochrane review found that the use of cleansers followed by leave-on moisturizers or protectants works better than soap and water to prevent skin inflammation. Avoid products with alcohol or propylene glycol, which can irritate the skin or cause an allergic reaction.

For more information, go to the website of the National Association for Continence at www.nafc.org.

Odor control

An unpleasant urine smell can interfere with your work and social activities. But simple changes in your normal routine can help.

If you don't drink much fluid, a strong odor may mean your urine is too concentrated. If so, drinking more water may help. But don't go overboard, or you might increase leakage. Acidic urine tends to have less odor, so you can take extra ascorbic acid (vitamin C) or cranberry juice to lower your urine's pH. Certain foods, such as asparagus, may add odor to the urine. A

---

strong odor to the urine may also be a sign of urinary tract infection.

Urine collection devices can be cleaned with plain white vinegar and water, and you can add vinegar or baking soda to your wash water to remove a urine smell from clothing. Vinegar is much better at eliminating odors than products that attempt to cover odors with heavy fragrances.

Emotional concerns

Whether your incontinence is mild or severe, you may be coping with a range of unpleasant emotions, including fear, embarrassment, anxiety, shame, and depression. Although you may feel quite isolated, help is available from many sources. Just getting medical treatment for incontinence has been shown to improve psychological well-being, whether or not the symptoms dramatically improve.

Consider seeking help from a therapist—particularly one familiar with incontinence. A therapist can help you cope with your emotions and with the rigors and uncertainties of treatment. And don't be afraid to tell your friends and family. You'd be surprised how many other people have experienced some form of incontinence. A support group can link you to others who are going through the same experience and can offer practical advice and emotional support. ▼

Fecal incontinence

Fecal incontinence is the unintended passage of stool. Both men and women may experience such leakage, but it is more common in women, particularly those who have given birth. For both men and women, fecal incontinence becomes more common with advancing age, as connective tissues and muscles of the pelvic floor weaken. According to the National Health and Nutrition Examination Survey, 6.8% of adult men and 10% of adult women reported experiencing the unintended leakage of stool within the previous month. The cost of dealing with fecal incontinence for an individual is estimated at more than $4,000 a year.

If you have fecal incontinence, you may not be able to hold in your stool long enough to reach the bathroom. Or you might experience unexpected leakage of stool when you haven't felt any urge (see Figure 8, below left). The symptoms of fecal incontinence can range from mild occasional leakage of liquid stool to a daily debilitating condition with consequences for self-confidence, self-image, and the ability to maintain friendships or careers. Most people with fecal incontinence don't tell their friends, families, or even their doctors. Instead, they limit their activities to avoid accidents and embarrassment. This can result in isolation and depression.

Because people are reluctant to seek help, fecal incontinence is sometimes perceived as rare. This perception is wrong. Even though people may not disclose it readily, fecal incontinence often goes hand in hand with urinary incontinence. It occurs in adults of all ages, and for older or disabled people, it is a leading reason for nursing home placement. One survey found that nearly half of nursing home residents had fecal incontinence.

Most people with fecal incontinence can be helped. If you or someone you know is experiencing fecal incontinence, seek medical advice. There are new options for evaluating, treating, and managing this distressing condition, and even if your previous attempts to get help have been unsatisfactory, you may be able to get help now. While available treatments may not completely cure fecal incontinence, they can lead to gradual improvements that increase quality of life and allow a patient to participate more fully in daily activities.

Anatomy of fecal continence

You rely on your digestive system to process the food you eat. The system absorbs vital nutrients into the bloodstream, and then removes the remaining waste products and indigestible food components from your body. By the time food has traveled through your

Figure 8: Causes of fecal incontinence

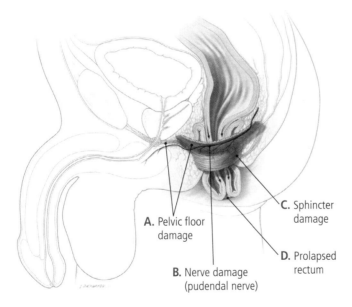

A. Pelvic floor damage

B. Nerve damage (pudendal nerve)

C. Sphincter damage

D. Prolapsed rectum

Surgery, constipation, and radiation treatments are among the factors that contribute to fecal incontinence. For example, surgery may cause damage to pelvic floor muscles (**A**), the pudendal nerve (**B**), or the anal sphincters (**C**). Chronic diarrhea or constipation can damage the rectum (**D**). In women, vaginal childbirth can also damage the anal sphincters, leading to fecal incontinence.

digestive tract to your large intestine, or colon, it is made up of waste material, which continues to lose water and solidify as it slowly moves along. The final product is known as stool, or feces.

At the end of your digestive tract are two areas crucial to fecal continence: the rectum and the anal canal. Muscles in the colon propel feces into the rectum, which has walls that stretch to hold the stool. The last inch of the rectum is called the anal canal. Two kinds of muscle surround it. The internal anal sphincter, which is not under your conscious control, stays contracted most of the time to prevent leakage. The external anal sphincter surrounds the internal anal sphincter.

How does your body know when to release stool? You have stretch-detecting nerve endings in the rectum. When your nerves detect that the rectum is full, the internal sphincter opens briefly and lets a tiny bit of the rectum's contents come in contact with the external sphincter, which is rich with nerve endings. In a rapid "sampling reflex," these nerves inform the brain about whether the rectal contents are intestinal gas or liquid or solid stool. This allows you to act accordingly. You might allow gas to escape, or look for a bathroom right away if you have diarrhea. Otherwise, you might decide whether it is convenient to have a bowel movement, or whether you want to wait for a better time or place.

To delay, you tighten the external anal sphincter (usually without thinking about it) to hold feces inside. As you are attempting to hold in stool, you also contract the puborectalis muscle, a pelvic floor muscle that loops around the rectum. When this muscle is contracted, it pulls the rectum so that it lies at a 90-degree angle to the anal canal rather than more directly above it. This counters the pull of gravity. Contracting these muscles often curbs the urge to defecate. The urge returns when more feces enter the rectum.

Once you are in the bathroom, you relax the puborectalis muscle and both the internal and external sphincters. Then, to propel the stool downward, you increase pressure in the abdominal cavity through the Valsalva or "bearing down" maneuver—closing off the airway, tightening the abdominal muscles, and pushing the diaphragm down.

What can go wrong?

Fecal incontinence is a symptom, not a disease. It can result if something goes wrong with any of the coordinated mechanisms that help maintain continence. The problem is not always caused by a malfunction in the gastrointestinal tract. In some situations, functional incontinence occurs when an unrelated condition, such as arthritis, makes it physically difficult to reach the toilet. In other situations, incontinence involves the malfunction of the bowel or rectum. This kind of incontinence usually stems from one of several common causes.

Bowel problems. Even if your rectum and anal canal are functioning properly, the system can be overwhelmed by conditions that speed the passage of waste products through the colon, resulting in diarrhea. For example, you may have incontinence temporarily during a bout of food poisoning or in reaction to a medication.

Conditions that cause chronic diarrhea, such as celiac disease, irritable bowel syndrome, and inflammatory bowel disease, can lead to occasional or ongoing problems with fecal incontinence. Diabetes may cause nighttime diarrhea that is difficult to control. Sometimes people with minor sphincter damage are able to maintain continence for a long time. But years after the damage, a bowel problem may develop that stresses the sphincters and ends their control.

Reduced rectal capacity. Surgery, pelvic radiation (to treat cancer of the prostate or uterus), or inflammatory bowel disease can stiffen or scar the rectum. Then the rectum loses elasticity and cannot store a normal amount of stool. You will have less time between the sensation of stool being present and an urgent need to find a toilet. Diarrhea is particularly difficult to hold.

Constipation. When hard fecal matter becomes stuck in the rectum, constipation or impaction may occur, causing liquid stool to eventually leak out around the hardened stool. This type of fecal incontinence is called overflow incontinence. It can be confused with diarrhea, but antidiarrheal medications only make the situation worse.

Sphincter damage. If the internal anal sphincter is damaged, bits of stool can leak out without you being aware of it or able to control it. This may occur at times of physical exertion or after you have had a bowel movement. If, on the other hand, the external anal sphincter muscles are damaged, you may be unable to squeeze hard enough or long enough to make it to the toilet. While you are rushing to the bathroom, fecal leakage may occur. In women, the most common cause of sphincter injury is vaginal childbirth. The risk increases if a woman has a large baby; is older; or has a long second stage of labor (pushing), a forceps delivery, a tear that extends to the anus, or an episiotomy (an incision to extend the vaginal opening in an attempt to avoid a tear). Sometimes fecal incontinence is apparent immediately after childbirth. Other times, when less severe sphincter damage occurs, symptoms of incontinence do not appear until decades later. The anal sphincters can also be damaged during rectal surgery (to treat prolapse, hemorrhoids, malformations, or rectal cancer), traumatic injury, or anal intercourse.

Pelvic floor muscle weakness and thinning. Fecal incontinence can result if your pelvic floor muscles become weak, or if they contract and relax at inappropriate times. Pelvic floor weakness might result from vaginal deliveries or years of straining to defecate.

Rectal prolapse. When the muscles supporting the rectum are weak, the rectal lining may descend into the anal canal or even protrude from the body. (Hemorrhoids are not rectal prolapse.) If you have a rectal prolapse, you may feel an urgent need to go even when little stool is present. Your external sphincter must work harder to keep you continent. Most people with rectal prolapse have some degree of fecal incontinence. Untreated rectal prolapse can cause long-term stretching and damage of the sphincter, so it is important to seek treatment if you notice any sign of rectal tissue emerging from the anus.

Nerve damage. If nerves controlling the sphincters malfunction, proper muscle action is impaired, and incontinence may develop. If sensory nerves are damaged, it becomes difficult to perceive that there is stool in the rectum. The pudendal nerve is the major nerve supplying the external sphincter. Damage to this nerve, resulting in incontinence, can occur when the pelvic floor muscles are stretched or traumatized

by childbirth or repeated straining to defecate, or if a person develops a neurological condition (such as multiple sclerosis, stroke, diabetic neuropathy, or spinal cord injury).

Rectocele. In women, the rectum may bulge into the vagina because of weakening of the vaginal wall. This can be caused by vaginal childbirth. Some women find it helps to place one or more fingers inside the vagina when having a bowel movement, to help support the bulging tissue. Rectocele is not considered to be a direct cause of fecal incontinence, but it is sometimes associated with intussusception, the first stage of rectal prolapse, which can cause either incontinence or constipation.

Evaluating fecal incontinence

A surprising number of people with fecal incontinence don't seek medical attention. Half of those with severe incontinence and 95% of people with occasional accidents try to cope on their own and therefore miss getting the help that is available. Your primary care physician is likely to be a good place to start, but don't be surprised if you are referred to a specialist for evaluation (see "Finding a clinician," page 11). Ideally, your physicians will work together to arrive at the best approach to the problem.

Talking to your doctor about fecal incontinence can be embarrassing. Keep in mind that, to your physician, fecal incontinence is not a personal problem, but a medical symptom like any other—one that needs to be investigated thoroughly because there are so many possible causes. To that end, you can help by being prepared to answer detailed questions:

- When did the incontinence start?
- How often do you have an accident? What happens? Do you lose a large or small amount of stool? Do you have any warning? Does anything seem to bring it on (such as physical activity, stress, time in menstrual cycle, particular foods)?
- Is it getting worse over time? Does anything seem to make it better or worse?
- When your rectum is full, can you distinguish whether it is solid, liquid, or gas? Do you sometimes think you are passing gas, only to be sur-

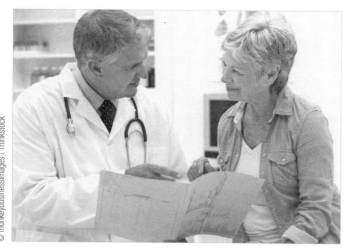

Nearly 7% of men and 10% of women have fecal incontinence. If you are one of them, don't suffer in silence. Today there are new options for evaluating, treating, and managing the condition.

prised that stool has come out?

- When you feel the need to have a bowel movement, how long can you wait?
- After you defecate, do you feel like there is stool left inside?
- What are your regular bowel habits? Do you often have diarrhea or constipation? Do you often have cramps or see blood in your stool?
- Are you using pads or other means to manage the incontinence? How is it working?
- Do you use any products to prevent constipation?
- Do you also experience urinary incontinence?

Because a wide variety of medical conditions and injuries can affect continence (and the symptoms may not appear until much later), the doctor will need a detailed medical history. If you have delivered one or more babies, it may be helpful to tell the doctor about the length of your labors, how much the babies weighed, whether deliveries involved the use of forceps or episiotomies, whether you had any tears that needed repair, and how your bowels functioned after the deliveries.

Let the physician know about other medical conditions you have and any medications (over-the-counter or prescription) you take. Also relevant are any injuries or treatments in your pelvic region. For example, have you had prostate or hemorrhoid surgery? Radiation to the pelvic area? An injury involving your spine or your anus?

Be frank about your concerns. Although fecal incontinence is rarely the first sign of rectal cancer or another serious medical condition, let your doctor know about your fears. And make sure the doctor knows exactly how the incontinence is affecting your life and how you are attempting to manage it. During your evaluation, your physician—or a nurse who specializes in incontinence—may be able to suggest more effective ways to manage the problem.

The physical exam

A physical examination is an important part of the diagnostic process. During the physical exam, your clinician will check your reflexes, walking gait, and senses for signs of general neurological disease or damage. He or she will also examine your abdomen for indications of bowel problems. The main difference you will notice between a standard physical and an evaluation for fecal incontinence is that the rectal exam is more thorough than usual.

First, the clinician looks at and inside the anus for any skin damage or scarring from previous injuries or medical procedures. The shape of your anus—whether open or closed, perfectly round or asymmetrical, intact or cracked—is noted. Using a cotton swab or pinprick, the doctor touches various points around your anus to see if it puckers up—a normal "winking" reflex.

Next, the doctor inserts a gloved finger into your rectum for the digital rectal exam to feel for the presence of hemorrhoids, growths, tears, protrusions, or scars. You may be asked to squeeze your muscles around the doctor's finger or to bear down as if you were straining to have a bowel movement. The doctor may be able to feel whether the puborectalis muscle in your pelvic floor is working to keep the colon and rectum at the proper angle. If you feel any pain during the exam, tell the physician.

Testing

In about one-third of people with fecal incontinence, the physical exam does not provide a definite diagnosis. In that case, your doctor may order various tests.

Laboratory tests

If the doctor suspects an infection is causing diarrhea, he or she may take a stool sample and have it cultured in the laboratory so it can be examined for bacteria or other microbes. Other laboratory tests may be used to rule out various conditions that can have fecal incontinence as a symptom.

Exams using scopes

The doctor may want to take a closer look at the area suspected of causing the problem. Using a viewing device, or scope, your physician can check for tumors, inflammation, prolapse, or other changes in the lining of your lower colon or rectum that might indicate damage to underlying nerves and muscles.

Flexible sigmoidoscopy. This test can be performed in your physician's office or in the hospital. You'll receive instructions in advance on how to clean out your bowels—usually by fasting and taking a laxative the night before the test and using an enema an hour or two before your appointment. The enema irrigates the rectum with a stimulant solution so you will clean all the feces out of your rectum prior to the exam. While you lie on your side, the doctor inserts a lubricated sigmoidoscope (a flexible scope about half an inch wide and two feet long) through your rectum into your colon. The scope has a light and video camera, along with mechanisms for adding air or washing the area to get a better view. The exam takes about 20 minutes.

Colonoscopy. Using this method, the doctor examines the full length of the colon. This method is often used to screen for colon polyps and other signs of colon cancer. The test requires sedation. It is usually not necessary for evaluating fecal incontinence, but it may be suggested if colorectal cancer is suspected or if screening might be advisable for other reasons.

Other scope exams. For an examination that does not include the colon, your physician may use a proctoscope to examine the rectum or an anoscope to view the anal canal only.

Other tests

Even if nothing is apparent on the clinical exam and you don't recall a difficult childbirth or other trau-
matic injury, your doctor may still suspect that your anal sphincters are damaged. The following tests can help determine whether that is the case.

Anorectal manometry. A doctor may use this test to measure the pressure inside your rectum and anal sphincters. After you have an enema, the clinician inserts into your rectum a small flexible tube (about the width of a rectal thermometer). The tube has a balloon at the end. As you rest, squeeze, and bear down, the pressure inside your rectum and inside each sphincter is recorded on a polygraph-like display. This testing helps the clinician assess the strength of your sphincters and determine whether they are relaxing and constricting at the proper times. The test is a little bit like urodynamic testing (see page 10) for urinary incontinence.

Endoanal ultrasound. This technique, also known as endoanal sonography, uses sound waves, rather than x-rays, to create images of the internal and external anal sphincters. Inserting a slim ultrasound probe into the anus, the physician should be able to see how your sphincter muscles move and determine whether any portions of the muscles are injured. It is important to distinguish incontinence caused by sphincter damage—which may be surgically repairable—from that caused by other muscle or nerve damage. Endoanal sonography can help distinguish who will benefit from surgery and who will best respond to nonsurgical approaches.

Anorectal electromyography (EMG). This test helps assess whether your muscles are contracting and relaxing appropriately. For anal sphincter EMG, the doctor inserts a small electrode-containing sponge into your anal canal. The sponge records electrical signals from the sphincter muscles as you squeeze and relax.

Pudendal nerve terminal motor latency. This technique helps assess whether your nerves are properly able to control the action of your anal sphincters. For a pudendal nerve study, the clinician does a digital rectal exam with a small electrode attached to his or her index finger. The doctor delivers a mild electrical current to the pudendal nerve and measures the amount of time it takes for the sphincter to contract in response to the current.

X-rays. Rarely, special x-rays may be taken to help evaluate the anatomy and functioning of your pelvic floor muscles and rectum, or to locate any obstruction in the colon. These exams go by different names: defecography, dynamic defecography, or evacuation proctography. Before your appointment, you clean out your colon as you would for flexible sigmoidoscopy. One hour before the exam, you may be asked to drink some barium solution.

Just before the exam, a technician will insert a substance with the consistency of stool that is visible on x-ray into your rectum. Then the technician takes x-ray video images as you cough, squeeze your buttocks, strain, and defecate on a special commode. This test may reveal abnormal positioning of the rectum or relaxation of sphincter muscles. The exam is not painful, but you may have an uncomfortable feeling of needing to have a bowel movement. ◆

Treating fecal incontinence

Fecal incontinence can be treated. It is up to you and your doctor to decide which treatment is best for you. Choices range from dietary changes and bowel training regimens to surgery. The approach you select will depend on the cause and severity of the condition. To help you gain the best possible control, physicians often recommend a combination of approaches. In most cases, treatment begins with nonsurgical options.

Diet and medication

The good news is that your diet can have a major impact on your bowel function by changing the consistency of the stool and the predictability of your bowel movements. That means there are potentially beneficial changes that you can make, such as eating more fiber or eliminating foods that irritate your system. Depending on your symptoms, your doctor may suggest dietary changes to improve bowel control or make your condition easier to manage.

Virtually everyone can derive some benefit from dietary changes. For example, people with sphincter problems can gain better control by taking steps to eliminate diarrhea. Symptoms of irritable bowel syndrome can be helped by identifying and eliminating specific irritating foods.

Controlling diarrhea

Diarrhea is a very common aggravating factor in fecal incontinence. If you tend to have loose stools, you may be able to make them firmer and easier to control by adding fiber to your diet or by taking a bulking agent or fiber supplement (see "Quick tip," page 41). High-fiber diets can be helpful for both constipation and diarrhea. Dietary fiber can absorb up to 30 times its weight in water. It produces formed but soft stools, and may "normalize" your bowels. Good sources of dietary fiber are bran cereals, uncooked fruits and vegetables, whole-grain breads and pasta, and brown rice.

Specific foods may trigger diarrhea in some people. The National Institute of Diabetes and Digestive and Kidney Diseases (NIDDK) has identified a number of foods you might try eliminating from your diet to see if your symptoms improve (see "Foods that may cause diarrhea," page 42).

In people with irritable bowel syndrome (IBS), a diet that cuts out certain carbohydrates is sometimes helpful in reducing diarrhea along with abdominal pain, gas, and bloating. The troublesome carbohydrates are sugar-like molecules called fermentable oligo-, di-, and monosaccharides and polyols (FODMAPs). They're found in a variety of foods, including milk, some fruits and vegetables, wheat, rye, high-fructose corn syrup, and artificial sweeteners. FODMAPs are poorly absorbed from the small intestine into the bloodstream. Instead, gut bacteria feed on them, creating the gas and bloating that's a hallmark of IBS. Because FODMAPs are present in many foods, some associated with health benefits, it is recommended that you work closely with a registered dietitian who is very familiar with the diet if you decide to try it. Often after several weeks on the diet, you can gradually start to eat certain FODMAPs.

Your physician may advise a change in the medications you take for other conditions, in case they are contributing to diarrhea and incontinence problems. For instance, the antidiabetic drug metformin (Glucophage) sometimes causes chronic diarrhea, long after you start taking the drug. Another example is orlistat (Xenical), a medication used to treat obesity, which acts by decreasing the absorption of fat from the digestive tract. Side effects may include several distressing bowel symptoms, including oily seepage from the rectum, fecal urgency, and, for a few people, fecal incontinence.

If food seems to move through your digestive system rapidly, your doctor may suggest an antidiarrheal medicine such as loperamide (Imodium) or diphenoxylate and atropine (Lomotil). This can solidify your stools and make them less frequent. Loperamide has the side benefit of increasing muscle tone in the internal anal sphincter, which can also help with incontinence. In a side-by-side comparison, both psyllium powder and loperamide reduced fecal incontinence and improved quality of life. Another medication, the tricyclic antidepressant amitriptyline (Elavil), also reduces the number of bowel movements. Some doctors have used it successfully to improve fecal incontinence, although the effectiveness of this treatment has not yet been confirmed in a controlled study.

Managing constipation

If your fecal incontinence is related to constipation, your health professional may suggest ways to train yourself to have regularly timed bowel movements. These may include increasing your fiber and fluid intake and using various stimuli (from a warm drink to an enema) to encourage a bowel movement at set times.

Pelvic muscle conditioning

Improving your pelvic muscle tone can help with fecal as well as urinary incontinence.

Pelvic floor exercises

Using exercise to strengthen the muscles of the pelvic floor, including the anal sphincters, is a commonly recommended treatment for people with fecal incontinence (see "Pelvic floor exercises," page 17). The studies evaluating the effectiveness of pelvic muscle training in treating fecal incontinence have shown inconsistent results. However, for people whose incontinence is less than severe and who prefer a self-help method to surgery, pelvic floor strengthening is worth trying. Combining this technique with dietary changes (to increase fiber) and adjustment in medications as needed may improve the likelihood of success. As with any muscle-strengthening program, pelvic muscle strength begins to diminish as soon as the exercises are discontinued.

Biofeedback

Biofeedback training can help fecal incontinence in two ways. First, it helps you strengthen and coordinate the action of your sphincter muscles. This can provide an effective way to help identify the correct muscles for pelvic floor exercises, helping you learn how to do the exercises correctly (see "Using biofeedback to learn pelvic floor exercises," page 18). Second, biofeedback can improve your ability to sense the presence of stool in the rectum.

If the biofeedback session is aimed at strengthening your pelvic muscles, the practitioner will insert a slim sensor into your rectum. (In women, it is sometimes placed in the vagina, or an additional sensor may be used there.) Other electrodes will be placed on your abdomen to help record muscle contractions there. A computer screen provides feedback about the strength of your contractions and about whether you are using the correct muscles.

If the biofeedback training is aimed at improving your ability to sense stool in the rectum, the practitioner will use anorectal manometry equipment to vary the pressure in your rectum. This is intended to increase the sensitivity of the rectum, which, in turn, helps some people to recognize the presence of stool before the situation becomes desperate.

Whether biofeedback will help in your particular case depends on the cause and severity of your incontinence and your ability to learn and practice the exercises. The improvements may only be modest. But biofeedback and exercise are so safe they are almost always recommended before more invasive treatments.

Electrical stimulation

Another form of biofeedback training uses electrical stimulation. As a part of this treatment, a small electrical current is delivered to the anal sphincter, in hopes of bulking up the muscles. Unlike other biofeedback methods, electrical stimulation does the work for you, producing much more muscle activity than people can accomplish themselves, even with standard biofeedback. There are several reports that suggest this may be of value. But, so far, there have been no controlled studies that have compared its effectiveness with that of standard biofeedback.

Surgical treatments

If you do require surgery, the exact approach will depend on the cause of your symptoms and your response to previous treatments. Some of these approaches have been around for years—although the techniques are always being modified and updated to improve results. Other approaches are more recent developments.

Sacral nerve stimulation

Sacral nerve stimulation is a minimally invasive approach with a low rate of medical complications. For this procedure, the surgeon inserts a kind of pacemaker to provide continuous electric stimulation to the anal sphincter to keep it closed. This technique has long been used for urinary incontinence (see "Sacral nerve stimulation," page 22). In 2011, the FDA approved the use of this procedure for fecal incontinence, too. In both urinary and fecal incontinence, the same sacral nerve is stimulated (the third). In one study of 76 people with severe fecal incontinence, five years after implantation of the device, 89% had at least a 50% improvement in their incontinence and 36% had no more fecal incontinence.

There are some downsides. According to reports to the FDA, within the first few years almost 20% of patients require an additional surgical procedure in order to address complications and keep the device working properly. As with a pacemaker, you will need to have the battery replaced every five years. Also, you cannot undergo MRI (with some precautions, a head

MRI is allowed), even if the battery is turned off.

Sacral nerve stimulation for fecal incontinence is covered by Medicare and many private insurers, although the private insurers often require a lengthy pre-authorization process and have many exclusions.

Overlapping sphincteroplasty

If your anal sphincter has been damaged—for example, during childbirth or anal surgery—your physician may suggest a sphincteroplasty to repair it. The external anal sphincter forms a ring around the anus. If there is a breach or interruption in the ring of muscle, you may not be able to close it tightly enough to keep stool in. During a sphincteroplasty, the surgeon will reattach the damaged ends and stitch them together to create a complete ring of muscle. This restores the anus to its proper shape. Sphincteroplasty has been used for decades and is the most common surgery used to treat fecal incontinence. It is very safe. However, the effectiveness of sphincteroplasty may vary for different kinds of patients. Therefore, careful evaluation before surgery is important.

While you are healing from sphincteroplasty, you may have discomfort, bruising, and swelling in the wound area. Wound infections sometimes happen after sphincteroplasty—as they do after all surgeries in the anorectal area. As with any surgery, you should be scrupulous in following your doctor's instructions on cleaning and caring for the wound.

Sphincteroplasty has been shown to be successful—at least initially—in up to 75% of patients with severe fecal incontinence. However, there have also been discouraging reports about deterioration in

---

Foods that may cause diarrhea

Try eliminating or reducing the foods listed below, doing so one at a time for several days each, to determine whether one of them might be causing diarrhea.

- alcohol
- caffeine
- cured or smoked meats
- dairy products
- fatty and greasy foods
- fruits
- spicy foods
- sweeteners (fructose; sorbitol, xylitol, mannitol, found in many diet drinks, fruit drinks, sugarless gum, and candies)

---

function over time. In two studies, about half of the patients who underwent this treatment said they were experiencing some urinary or fecal incontinence, had required further surgery, or had developed other bowel problems, when contacted four to 12 years later. Results are better when patients are younger and less time has elapsed since the initial sphincter injury. In a small study comparing similar patients with sphincter defects, those treated with sacral nerve stimulation improved significantly more than those who underwent sphincteroplasty.

If incontinence is still a problem after the surgery, your surgeon may recommend additional biofeedback. In fact, some surgeons suggest it for all patients as soon as the wound is healed, in order to maximize the chance of a good outcome. Your physician may also suggest that you be checked for an injury to a rectal muscle called the levator ani, which may explain the persistence of symptoms. So far, however, there is no surgery to repair this type of injury.

Rectal prolapse repair

One common cause of fecal incontinence is rectal prolapse (also known as internal rectal intussusception)—the dropping of the rectum because of muscle weakness. If it is not treated, this condition can cause permanent damage to the sphincter. If it is surgically repaired, however, fecal incontinence may become much less severe, and, in many cases, it will be entirely cured. This surgery is most successful if done early, so don't put off reporting your symptoms to your doctor.

There are a variety of surgical options for treating rectal prolapse. The particular option that you are offered will depend in part upon your health. In general, younger, healthier patients will be offered an operation that involves an abdominal incision and removal of part of the bowel. This surgery can be done either through a traditional open incision or by using laparoscopy (a camera-aided surgery that uses small surgical tools inserted through small incisions). In general, older patients will be offered a simpler surgery, through the anus. In this case, the protruding rectal tissue will simply be cut off, so it does not stretch the anal sphincter. Both surgeries work well in the short term. However, an abdominal approach is generally preferable, if possible, because it lasts longer.

Artificial sphincter

Until recently, an artificial bowel sphincter was a surgical option available in the United States for patients whose severe sphincter injury is beyond repair or does not respond to other surgery. The doctor inserted an artificial device that circled the anal sphincter. It kept the anus closed until the patient squeezed a control pump to open it. The opening, in turn, allowed a bowel movement to pass. Afterward, the cuff gradually closed. For a male patient, the control pump was implanted in the scrotum. For a female patient, it was inserted in one of the labia.

In follow-up studies, the implantation of an artificial sphincter cured fecal incontinence and significantly improved quality of life in most patients. But some patients required repeat surgery or had complications, such as infection; these patients had to have the device removed.

By 2017, the company that made the artificial sphincter had discontinued manufacturing the device, and without this option, more patients with severe sphincter injury may undergo colostomy (see page 44).

Magnetic sphincter augmentation

Between 2015 and 2017, an alternative to the artificial sphincter, magnetic sphincter augmentation (the FENIX continence restoration system), was available as a treatment of last resort if other surgery failed. It used a flexible band of titanium beads with magnetic cores. The band was wrapped around the anal sphincter in a surgical procedure. The magnetic attraction between the beads was designed to hold the sphincter closed, except to allow defecation. The device was adapted from a successful approach to gastroesophageal reflux disease, the Linx procedure, which was approved by the FDA in 2012.

Sales and clinical studies of the device were stopped by the manufacturer in 2017, although support continues to be available to those who already have the device. Without this option, more patients may undergo colostomy (see page 44).

Antegrade colonic enema surgery

When other techniques have not been successful, you can opt for a surgical procedure to create a small opening (stoma) on the side of the abdomen that allows you to empty your bowels on a routine schedule. During the procedure, a small passageway is created between the skin of the abdomen and the colon, using a section of small intestine as the tube (called a cecostomy tube). Afterward, to empty your bowels, you sit on the toilet and insert fluid through the stoma, allowing the fluid and feces to flow out through the anus. Flushing the bowels until empty usually takes 30 to 60 minutes. In many cases, this surgery can be performed laparoscopically.

Colostomy

A final surgical technique—usually done as a last resort—is colostomy. This means that feces are entirely diverted from the rectum and anal canal and instead leave the body through a surgically created opening. In a colostomy, the surgeon attaches the end of the bowel to an opening made in your abdomen. The surgery is performed under general anesthesia and requires several days of hospitalization.

After a colostomy, you will need to care for the opening on the skin (called the ostomy), and you will need to wear a small pouch outside your body to collect waste material. Modern ostomy bags are not visible when you are dressed, and they control odor very effectively. Most of the time, no one is even aware that you have had the surgery.

Injection of bulking agents

Thus far, the injection of bulking agents to tighten the sphincter has not seen the success that had been hoped for. Injected into tissue layers of the anal canal, a gel containing small beads thickens the canal with the goal of keeping it closed. In a controlled trial of hyaluronic acid/dextranomer (Solesta), the only agent approved for this use in the United States, 53% of patients who received injections of the bulking agent achieved at least a 50% reduction in episodes of fecal incontinence, compared with 30.7% of patients who received sham injections. The procedure is simple and is usually done in an office setting. The injections are used in selected patients who have not responded to conservative therapies and who recognize they may only achieve moderate improvement. Its effectiveness, particularly over the long term, has not met expectations. In one study, after seven years, only 14% of the bulking agent was detectable on ultrasound, and it was no longer effective in treating incontinence. ▼

Coping with fecal incontinence

Even if treatment doesn't fully alleviate your symptoms, it is likely to diminish them and make your condition more manageable. Seek help from health professionals, such as continence nurses, and support organizations, such as the International Foundation for Functional Gastrointestinal Disorders (see "Resources," page 47). You can reclaim a sense of control by learning some coping strategies.

Skin care

When the skin comes in contact with fecal material for a length of time, it can become irritated and inflamed. That means proper care of the skin in the anal area is essential to maintaining comfort and preventing skin deterioration. Skin irritation is more than a misery. It can invite infection and even compromise your treatment if the skin becomes too sore for your muscles to work well. If you have both urinary and fecal incontinence, bacteria in the feces can react with urine to produce ammonia, which lowers the skin pH and leaves it more vulnerable to infection. Yeast infections can also develop, when yeast in the feces is nurtured by contact with urine.

Skin should be cleansed after each episode of incontinence. Choose an extremely mild, nonalkaline soap—such as Dove or Basis—or buy one of the special cleansers designed to gently dissolve and remove stool and urine (such as Aplicare Antiseptic Perineal Wash). These are nonirritating, soap-free cleansing lotions; some are available in portable disposable wipes (Clinell Continence Care Wipes). They eliminate the need to scrub areas of tender skin, and some do not require that you rinse the skin after use. In studies conducted in nursing homes, the cleansers worked better than soap to prevent breakdown of sensitive perineal skin in patients with incontinence.

After cleansing, allow the area to air-dry if possible, or blow dry with a hair dryer set on cool, or pat it dry (don't rub). Afterward, apply a protective moisturizer or moisture barrier to protect the skin from damage by urine or stool contact. Barrier products such as petroleum jelly, Aquaphor, and Desitin are readily available and inexpensive.

Film-forming skin protectants (Cutimed Protect, 3M Cavilon No Sting Barrier Film)—applied by spray, applicator, or individual wipe—go on as a liquid but rapidly evaporate. They leave behind a film of clear acrylate. This barrier allows airflow, but protects the skin from moisture. Film-forming skin protectants may help reduce the rubbing of pads or absorbent products or make it less irritating to use products applied with adhesive. Some films last as long as three days before reapplication is needed.

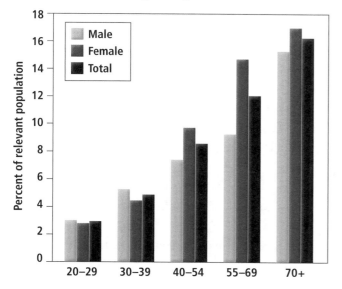

Figure 9: Prevalence of fecal incontinence according to age and sex

Fecal incontinence is somewhat more common in women than in men, but in both genders, the most noticeable trend is that prevalence climbs steeply with age.

Reprinted with permission from Ditah I, et al. "Prevalence, trends, and risk factors for fecal incontinence in United States adults, 2005–2010," Clinical Gastroenterology and Hepatology (April 2014), Vol. 12, No. 4, pp. 636–43.

To treat or protect against fungal infection, you may be instructed to use an ointment or cream containing an antifungal agent, such as clotrimazole or miconazole. Ask whether you should apply another barrier product while using the antifungal.

A nurse who deals with incontinence or stoma care can offer advice on skin care issues. For more information, go to the website of the National Association for Continence at www.nafc.org.

Reducing odor

Minimizing the odor of stool can make leakage less noticeable to yourself and others. Dietary changes can help by eliminating foods that commonly increase stool odor. Such foods include fish, eggs, asparagus, garlic, cruciferous vegetables (such as cabbage, broccoli, and cauliflower), onions, beans, and turnips.

Odor can also be reduced by taking an internal deodorant containing chlorophyllin copper (such as Nullo) or bismuth subgallate (such as Devrom). Both are available without prescription. However, chlorophyllin may color your urine and stool green. This creates the possibility of "grass-stained" clothing if an accident occurs. If cramping or diarrhea occurs when taking chlorophyllin, reduce the dose. If symptoms continue, stop taking it.

Containment and collection options

Absorbent products, such as pads and disposable undergarments, are designed primarily for urinary incontinence, and people with fecal incontinence often find them unsatisfactory. Of the range of choices available, those that provide "heavy" protection are most likely to be helpful for fecal incontinence. According to the limited studies available, disposable products with super-absorbent materials may provide the best protection and be easiest on your skin.

There are also fecal collection devices (such as Bard FCD and Hollister Fecal Collectors), which are pouches that adhere to the skin around the anus to collect uncontrolled stool leakage. These devices control stool odor and can drain off liquid into a separate bag. You can order such products through a medical supply house or catalog.

Enemas and suppositories

Some people with fecal incontinence are able to eliminate or minimize incontinence or soiling by using enemas or suppositories each morning to cleanse feces from their rectum and lower colon. Before using this self-treatment approach, you should get a medical evaluation to rule out serious conditions (such as cancer) and to obtain advice about possible side effects and the choice of an enema or suppository.

Emotional concerns

Gaining control over fecal incontinence is a psychological as well as physical challenge. The emotional repercussions can be very difficult to handle. You may find it helpful to remind yourself that this is a very common medical condition. Many other people, like you, are coping with the same condition, as the result of surgery, childbirth, or illness.

If you have lived with the problem for a long time before seeking help, it may take time and professional support for you to address your painful feelings and regain confidence in your ability to fully participate in normal activities and relationships.

Help is available from health professionals, therapists, and support groups. You can benefit greatly from the advice and experiences of others with the same problem, whether through informal contact or a support group. Most importantly, remember that this is a medical condition, not a personal weakness. ◆

Resources

Organizations

American Physical Therapy Association
1111 N. Fairfax St.
Alexandria, VA 22314
800-999-2782 (toll-free)
www.apta.org and www.womenshealthapta.org/pt-locator

This organization's locator can help you find a physical therapist specializing in urinary or bowel incontinence.

American Society of Colon and Rectal Surgeons
85 W. Algonquin Road, Suite 550
Arlington Heights, IL 60005
847-290-9184
www.fascrs.org

This professional society offers educational materials on fecal incontinence and many bowel-related tests and procedures. The website includes a locator for certified colorectal surgeons.

American Urogynecologic Society
1100 Wayne Ave., Suite 670
Silver Spring, MD 20910
301-273-0570
www.voicesforpfd.org

This professional society offers educational materials on incontinence for consumers and professionals. The website includes a locator for member urogynecologists, nurse practitioners, and physical therapists specializing in pelvic floor disorders, as well as a community blog and a chat room where you can pose questions to a urogynecologist.

American Urological Association
1000 Corporate Blvd.
Linthicum, MD 21090
866-746-4282 (toll-free)
www.urologyhealth.org

This professional society provides patient information on urologic disease and a doctor-locator function on its website.

Biofeedback Certification International Alliance
5310 Ward Road, Suite 201
Arvada, CO 80002
702-502-5829
www.bcia.org

The website for this organization can help you identify certified biofeedback practitioners in your area, including those certified to treat elimination disorders and pelvic pain.

International Foundation for Functional Gastrointestinal Disorders
P.O. Box 170864
Milwaukee, WI 53217
414-964-1799
www.aboutincontinence.org

The website for this organization provides a physician locator along with information and support for people dealing with fecal incontinence and other chronic digestive problems.

National Association for Continence
P.O. Box 1019
Charleston, SC 29402
800-252-3337 (toll-free)
www.nafc.org

The largest consumer advocacy and educational organization dealing with incontinence, NAFC provides a wide range of pamphlets and other materials, including a detailed brand-name resource guide to products, devices, and medications used to maintain an active life while coping with incontinence.

Wound, Ostomy, and Continence Nurses Society
1120 Route 73, Suite 200
Mt. Laurel, NJ 08054
888-224-9626 (toll-free)
www.wocn.org

Many members of this professional society specialize in the management and treatment of urinary and fecal incontinence and related conditions.

Books

The Bathroom Key: Put an End to Incontinence
Katherine Kassai, P.T., and Kim Perelli
(Demos Health, 2011)

This easy-to-read, illustrated book focuses on home programs to treat urinary incontinence and pelvic organ prolapse using physical therapy techniques.

Managing Life with Incontinence
Cheryle B. Gartley, Mary Radtke Klein, Christine Norton, Ph.D., R.N., and Anita Saltmarche, R.N., B.Sc.N., M.H.Sc.
(Simon Foundation for Continence, 2012)

Drawing on the experiences of patients and international incontinence experts, this book provides practical advice on managing urinary and fecal incontinence while improving your quality of life.

Regaining Bladder Control: What Every Woman Needs to Know
Rebecca G. Rogers, M.D., Janet Yagoda Shagam, Ph.D., and Shelley Kleinschmidt
(Prometheus Books, 2006)

Although a decade old, this book still provides useful supportive and practical information about getting help for urinary incontinence. Written by a urogynecologist in collaboration with medical writers, it includes at-home techniques to try, several worksheets, questions to ask, and clear illustrations and photographs. There are chapters on fecal incontinence and prolapse.

Harvard Special Health Reports

The following reports can be ordered by calling 877-649-9457 (toll-free) or online at www.health.harvard.edu.

A Guide to Men's Health: Fifty and forward
Anthony L. Komaroff, M.D., Medical Editor
(Harvard Medical School, 2016)

An overview of health issues that become more common as men pass age 50, with sections on reducing the risks for major diseases and tackling disorders before they become disabling.

A Guide to Women's Health: Fifty and forward
Hope Ricciotti, M.D., Medical Editor
(Harvard Medical School, 2016)

An overview of health issues for women past the age of 50, including sections on pelvic organ prolapse and persistent menopausal symptoms.

2017 Annual Report on Prostate Diseases
Marc B. Garnick, M.D., Medical Editor
(Harvard Medical School, 2017)

This report discusses advances in the diagnosis and treatment of prostate cancer, benign prostatic hyperplasia, prostatitis, erectile dysfunction, and related issues, including urinary incontinence.

The Sensitive Gut: A guide to managing common gastrointestinal disorders
Lawrence S. Friedman, M.D., Medical Editor
(Harvard Medical School, 2015)

This report covers a variety of GI conditions, including reflux, irritable bowel syndrome, constipation, and diarrhea.